Praise for

AWAKENED SLEEP

"*Awakened Sleep* is a lively and knowledgeable guide to improving health and well-being through proper sleep routines as well as a galvanizing call to experience sleep as a gateway to higher states of consciousness."

—Anand Dhruva, MD, professor of medicine, Osher Foundation Endowed Chair in Education in Integrative Health, director of education at the UCSF Osher Center for Integrative Health, associate program director of the Hematology Oncology Clinical Fellowship, Division of Hematology and Oncology, University of California, San Francisco

"In *Awakened Sleep*, Dr. Suhas Kshirsagar and Dr. Sheila Patel present a groundbreaking approach to restorative sleep. This comprehensive guide transforms our understanding of sleep, offering practical insights to help readers achieve the rest they need. As renowned practitioners with extensive experience, Kshirsagar and Patel skillfully convey how Ayurvedic principles and consciousness can revolutionize sleep management. Reading this book has been a transformative experience, and has improved my own sleep quality!"

—Eddie Stern, MSc, CYT, author of *One Simple Thing: A New Look at the Science of Yoga and How It Can Transform Your Life*

"Dr. Patel is a leader in Ayurvedic medicine. Her wisdom is healing. Her knowledge leads to health transformation. This book is a culmination of years of study and practice and will help readers use Ayurvedic knowledge to improve their sleep and their lives."

—Mimi Guarneri, MD, FACC, president of Academy of Integrative Health and Medicine, medical director at Guarneri Integrative Health

"Dr. Suhas is quite the authentic Ayurvedic clinician and physician. This is a wonderful book from his own spiritual experiences of healing the body, mind, and spirit. This book, *Awakened Sleep*, will truly awaken the inner healer."   —Vasant Lad, BAM&S, MASc

"*Awakened Sleep* is a compelling reminder that sleep isn't just a shutdown—it's a return to the source of our purest potential. With equal parts practical guidance and timeless wisdom, Dr. Suhas and Dr. Patel offer an essential guide for a culture that urgently needs to awaken to the power of deep rest."

—Sarah Platt-Finger, cofounder of ISHTA Yoga and director of Chopra Yoga

"*Awakened Sleep* by Drs. Suhas and Patel expertly blends education with practical action, Western science with Ayurvedic texts and the physical, emotional, and spiritual aspects of sleep to get us motivated and prepared to enjoy our most restorative and rejuvenating sleep of our lives. By learning our optimal schedule based on our own constitution, we can take the science-backed recommendations to optimize our sleep and our lives."

—Melanie Fiorella, MD, DipACLM, director, Center for Integrative Medicine UCSD Healthcare

"This book is overdue in our sleep deprived world. The authors, with their vast learning and experience in Ayurveda, have given us insights and practical advice on better living through better sleep."

—Swami Sarvapriyananda, spiritual leader, Vedanta Society of New York

AWAKENED
SLEEP

An AYURVEDIC APPROACH *to*
GETTING DEEP REST *and*
UNLOCKING OPTIMAL HEALTH

AWAKENED
SLEEP

SUHAS KSHIRSAGAR, BAMS, MD,
and SHEILA PATEL, MD

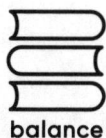

balance

New York   Boston

Balance

Hachette Book Group

1290 Avenue of the Americas

New York, NY 10104

GCP-Balance.com

@GCPBalance

First Edition: October 2025

Balance is an imprint of Grand Central Publishing. The Balance name and logo are registered trademarks of Hachette Book Group, Inc.

The publisher is not responsible for websites (or their content) that are not owned by the publisher.

Balance books may be purchased in bulk for business, educational, or promotional use. For information, please contact your local bookseller or the Hachette Book Group Special Markets Department at special.markets@hbgusa.com.

Print book interior design by Amy Quinn.

Library of Congress Cataloging-in-Publication Data

Names: Kshirsagar, Suhas G. author | Patel, Sheila (Holistic physician) author
Title: Awakened sleep : an Ayurvedic approach to getting deep rest and
    unlocking optimal health / Suhas Kshirsagar BAMS, MD and Sheila Patel, MD.
Description: First edition. | New York, NY : Balance, 2025. | Includes index.
Identifiers: LCCN 2025016804 | ISBN 9781538769317 hardcover |
    ISBN 9781538769331 ebook
Subjects: LCSH: Sleep disorders—Ayurvedic treatment | Medicine, Ayurvedic |
    Sleep | Sleep disorders—Alternative treatment | Holistic medicine | Self-care, Health
Classification: LCC RA786 .K795 2025
LC record available at https://lccn.loc.gov/2025016804

ISBNs: 9781538769317 (hardcover), 9781538769331 (ebook)

Printed in the United States of America

LSC-C

Printing 1, 2025

To our sleepless patients and students and to everyone who wants to awaken the healing potential of sleep

CONTENTS

FOREWORD

Dr. Deepak Chopra

I
N HUMAN EXISTENCE, SLEEP STANDS AS A PROFOUND MYSTERY—A UNI-
versal yet deeply personal phenomenon that bridges the worlds of the
seen and unseen. For millennia, sages and seekers have revered sleep as
more than a biological necessity; it is a sacred gateway to rejuvenation,
creativity, and spiritual awakening. In our modern world, dominated by
ceaseless activity and external distractions, sleep has become an elusive
treasure. Yet within each of us lies the innate potential to rediscover sleep,
not just as rest, but as a conscious journey into the infinite.

In the Vedic tradition, sleep is considered one of the three pillars of
health, alongside diet and mindful living. It is not merely the absence
of wakefulness but a state of profound recalibration, where body, mind,
and spirit align. Science, too, is beginning to glimpse this truth, revealing
that sleep is a cornerstone of our well-being, influencing everything from
physical vitality to emotional balance and spiritual clarity. But science
often stops at the mechanics of sleep, measuring its stages and cycles. To
truly awaken to the transformative power of sleep, we must move beyond
the clinical and embrace its essence as a portal to higher consciousness.

Awakened Sleep is a comprehensive manual for awakening consciousness through the powerful portal of sleep, offering a holistic approach
that honors both ancient wisdom and modern science. As we explore

this journey, it is important to acknowledge the challenges of our age. The demands of modern life—constant connectivity, artificial environments, and the glorification of busyness—have severed us from the natural rhythms that govern our biology. Sleep disorders, from insomnia to chronic fatigue, have become epidemic, affecting millions worldwide. The symptoms are familiar: fatigue, irritability, brain fog, and a diminished sense of joy. These are not just signs of a restless night; they are whispers from our deeper selves, urging us to return to balance.

This book is a bridge between ancient wisdom and modern insights, offering practical tools to reclaim the gifts of our circadian rhythm and experience "awakened sleep." This state transcends the basic function of rest, inviting us into a realm of expanded awareness where healing, intuition, and transformation become possible. It is the sleep of sages—a state of rest imbued with wakeful presence and spiritual insight.

To embark on this path, we must first understand the essence of sleep through three lenses: physical, mental/emotional, and spiritual well-being. Physically, sleep is the body's master healer, repairing tissues, strengthening immunity, and regulating our biological clocks. Mentally, it clears the mind, integrating memories and emotional experiences. Spiritually, it offers a rare opportunity to dissolve into the field of infinite possibilities, accessing the unbounded source of creativity and wisdom.

The journey to awakened sleep begins with awareness. How do you prepare for sleep? Are your evenings filled with overstimulation—bright screens, hurried meals, unresolved emotions? Or do you consciously create an environment of tranquility, signaling your body and mind to let go? These simple yet profound choices set the stage for the quality of sleep you will experience and, by extension, the life you will live.

Dr. Suhas Kshirsagar and Dr. Sheila Patel are your trusted guides on this journey. I have watched and worked closely with them both over the last two decades, and they are exceptional teachers and healers. Dr. Suhas is one of the most prominent Ayurvedic physicians in the world; he blends his clinical experience and knowledge in ways that are easy for a variety of audiences to digest and implement, in both his books and his teachings. As the medical director at the Chopra Center for Well-Being and then as the chief medical officer at Chopra Global for more than a decade, Dr. Sheila's knowledge of Ayurveda, meditation, and yoga is a powerful complement to her perspective on the latest medical and scientific findings. I have witnessed both of their regular teachings in our various Chopra programs, so I know firsthand that they accurately convey the intertwined messages of science and consciousness in ways that invite transformation. Indeed, *Awakened Sleep* captures the very essence of our collective teachings over the last forty years.

As you navigate these pages, you will encounter practical guidance rooted in the timeless principles of Ayurveda, the science of life. You will learn to harmonize your unique mind–body constitution, or *dosha*, with daily and seasonal rhythms. You will discover the transformative power of meditation and mindfulness, both as a prelude to sleep and as a way to enhance the quality of your dreams. And you will be introduced to the art of intentional rest, where you can plant the seeds of healing, creativity, and self-realization.

Awakened sleep is not a destination but a dynamic process—a dance between effort and surrender. It requires us to cultivate habits of alignment during our waking hours, as these are the moments that shape our nights. By attuning to the cycles of nature, embracing a diet of nourishing foods, engaging in mindful movement, and prioritizing emotional balance, we lay the foundation for restful and rejuvenating sleep.

One of the great paradoxes of awakened sleep is that it invites us to be both fully present and profoundly detached. As we drift into slumber, we release the identities and narratives that bind us to the waking world, entering a state of pure awareness. Here, in the silence of sleep, we reconnect with our true nature—unbounded, eternal, and blissful.

In sharing the wisdom of awakened sleep, we honor the union of science and spirit. Advances in neuroscience reveal how sleep orchestrates a symphony of processes, from synaptic pruning to hormonal balance. Simultaneously, spiritual traditions remind us that sleep is a sacred practice, a time to connect with the divine intelligence that sustains all life. By integrating these perspectives, we unlock the potential not only to sleep better but to live more fully.

Let this book be your guide, offering both inspiration and actionable steps to transform your relationship with sleep. Whether you struggle with insomnia, yearn for greater vitality, or seek deeper spiritual connection, the practices within these pages are designed to meet you where you are and take you where you wish to go. Through the lens of awakened sleep, every night becomes an opportunity to heal, grow, and awaken to the infinite possibilities of your being.

As you embark on this journey, remember that the essence of sleep is not found in striving but in surrender. Trust in the wisdom of your body, the rhythm of the cosmos, and the boundless field of consciousness that unites us all. In this state of awakened sleep, you will rediscover the truth of who you are: a luminous, eternal being, ever connected to the infinite.

INTRODUCTION

> What all beings consider as day is the night of
> ignorance for the Wise, and what all creatures see as
> night is the day for the fully awake introspective Sage.
>
> —*Bhagavad Gita*, Chapter 2:69

SLEEP IS A MIRACLE CURE THAT OPTIMIZES ALL OUR FUNCTIONS. IT'S an untapped source of physical, mental, and spiritual well-being that may very well hold the secrets to the universe—and to our capacity for deep, sustainable joy.

Yet we're not using this incredible tool to its full potential. Sleep is as important to our health as air, water, and food, yet it is often ignored until we feel the effects of poor sleep. If you've found your way to this book, you likely already know that ours is a sleep-deprived culture. One in three adults worldwide suffers from insomnia. With the increasingly hectic pace of our daily lives, compounded by the prevalence of gadgets, machines, and screens, it's little wonder that few of us are getting restorative sleep—which gives us robust physical and mental health, peace, longevity, and access to our full creative potential.

So many of us walk around with the negative effects that come with lack of sleep—dysregulated moods, fatigue, and a persistent mental fog—yet we somehow find a way to power through and become accustomed to feeling this way. Modern environmental challenges like increased artificial light exposure affect our natural rhythms. We're no longer aligned with the light and dark cycles in the same ways our ancestors were.

Insufficient sleep takes a significant toll on our health. In 2023 alone, there were twenty-four thousand articles written about sleep. Millions of Google searches include the word *sleep*, and in 2023, that number reached an all-time high. It's likely that none of this will come as news to you—and based on the statistics, it's also likely that finding the right solution to poor sleep can feel like trying to pluck the proverbial needle from the haystack. Often, even when practicing good sleep hygiene, we still don't wake up feeling rested. Our busy lifestyles and erratic routines place little value on the power of rest to rejuvenate our bodies, minds, and spirits and improve our moods, relationships, health, and overall happiness.

Sleep issues affect people of all ages. Indeed, restful sleep becomes more challenging as we age, but children are also struggling to get good sleep. The postpandemic "new normal" of working from home has made it doubly challenging for people to leave work at the office, contributing to more stress and a lack of balance—which can lead to an undue amount of tossing and turning and missing hours of sleep we'll never regain. According to a recent Gallup poll, only 39 percent of millennials reported getting enough sleep, while only 55 percent of people over age fifty-five felt satisfied with their sleep.[1] If time is money, millennials are broke.

Although clinicians and patients alike recognize the importance of sleep, a 2023 large-scale survey of Americans with trouble sleeping reported that 30 percent of these patients were not asked about sleep by their primary care provider, and two-thirds of those surveyed did not feel current treatment options adequately improved their sleep.[2]

A lot of us say we're looking for a good night's sleep, but how many of us actually know what that means? And how many of us know *how* to have it—or can identify the factors that are contributing to its lack?

YOUR NATURAL STATE

Thankfully, we all have the capacity for **awakened sleep**. **This enlightened, natural state allows us to wake up from the sleep of ignorance so that we can slumber in a restful awareness and create better health and self-regenerating happiness.**

Awakened sleep gradually allows us to have optimal energy, superior cognition and brain functioning, more balanced emotions, and greater longevity—especially when compared to the average person's sleep, which is generally accompanied by fitful dreams, tossing and turning, and feeling tired the next day despite clocking the "correct" number of hours.

Awakened sleep goes beyond physiological rest and relaxation, which is how most people frame good sleep. We know we need sleep to harness our body's natural restorative functions, but sleep has also been revered as an important mystical experience since time immemorial. Throughout the millennia, sages and scholars have had the understanding that it's possible to manifest miracles in our sleep, during which messages filter through our subconscious as unbridled creativity, unimpeded by the hustle and bustle of our daily lives. Awakened sleep gives us ready access to the wide-open field of consciousness and pure potential that we fail to access on a daily basis, both while awake and while asleep. In fact, awakened sleep holds the keys to the health of our body, mind, and spirit.

We're writing this book because we believe everyone has the right to access this field. *Awakened Sleep: An Ayurvedic Approach to Getting Deep Rest and Unlocking Optimal Health* is informed by our five combined decades of clinical practice and research. In our individual clinical practices and our collaborative work with Chopra Global, we fuse our deep knowledge of Western and Eastern medical approaches. We integrate cutting-edge scientific research with timeless practices to help people create balanced, restorative sleep that can unlock their full human potential. Through our work with thousands of patients and clients across the world, we have both been sharing conventional and holistic medical wisdom that has transformed lives, including our own, and assisted many in improving their health, and sleep, in practical and effective ways.

This book is our attempt to bridge the gap between modern science and ancient wisdom traditions so that you can improve your life on every level and be empowered to take control of your health and well-being.

Our aim is to offer you a holistic solution to a widespread problem, with a different approach than the majority of the sleep manuals you've read on your quest for good sleep. We offer new perspectives that can help you create a personalized sleep plan that's specific to you. But beyond improving your sleep, we hope this book will be a starting point for gaining deeper peace and meaning from your daily habits and practices.

Awakened Sleep is especially for you if you've ever faced the following:

- an ongoing struggle when it comes to getting enough sleep or quality sleep
- the need to resort to sleep aids, including medications and natural supplements, to combat sleepless nights
- the feeling of being physically or mentally "low" and knowing deep down that sleep is the problem (and the solution)
- the desire to use your sleeping hours to access more creativity and to manifest your intentions
- curiosity about how you might expand your meditative practice and understanding of sleep from a higher perspective—one that goes beyond your body's needs and into the needs of your spirit

If any of this resonates with you, you're in good hands! We'll begin by discussing some of the practical considerations of sleep. We'll describe awakened sleep in depth, including information about the most common culprits that interfere with our natural sleep patterns and cycles.

Aside from offering insight into the Western scientific understanding of sleep, we'll look at sleep through an Ayurvedic lens. Ayurveda, literally translated as the "science of life," is a traditional healing system rooted in ancient Indian teachings that promotes a natural, holistic framework for understanding and optimizing our physical, mental, and spiritual health through aligning our lifestyle with the rhythms of nature.

We also discuss the implications of the absence of natural, restorative sleep—and how this can impair your overall well-being in the long term. Throughout this section, we'll be weaving in three fundamental pillars of well-being—physical, mental/emotional, and spiritual—that affect our lives in various ways. We'll talk about what happens to our overall well-being when we sleep and how compromising sleep can disrupt every aspect of our health—sometimes, in unexpected ways. You'll start to reflect on your unique circumstances and become more conscious of how your sleep might be affecting the three pillars of your well-being.

In Part 2, we'll share the emotional and spiritual aspects that help us tap into awakened sleep. We'll discuss the power of your senses in establishing awakened sleep—beyond utilizing your physical senses for greater relaxation, you'll gain an awareness of the stimuli that may be lingering in your consciousness as you fall asleep. We'll also dig into how to soothe your nervous systems in the wake of trauma and other emotional experiences that may disrupt your sleep and disconnect you from your full vitality. We'll then segue into the more metaphysical aspects of sleep, describing them from a Vedic perspective. Vedic philosophy hails from the Vedas, a set of wisdom treatises from ancient India that are thousands of years old and widely believed to be the oldest texts detailing the metaphysics of the entire universe and functioning as a basis for how we can lead spiritually and materially fulfilling lives. The medical system of Ayurveda is rooted in Vedic philosophy and can help to fill in the informational gaps for which science hasn't been able to provide explanations. We'll delve into the magical, mind-bending world of dreams, where we can play with our fundamental beliefs about reality and reprogram ourselves to experience awakened sleep and a more fulfilling waking life. We'll also discuss yogic and meditative techniques that enable us to make sleep an extension of our spiritual practice. An integral aspect of total well-being is a deeper connection to what we might call the "divine"— the sense of peace within us that passes understanding, allows us to explore our full potential, and helps us to actively participate in and create a more grounded and beautiful waking reality.

The final section brings together the sleep protocols and tips you'll find throughout the book, so you can craft your own morning and evening rituals for awakened sleep. The insight you'll gain in Parts 1 and 2— through assessments, meditations, practices, and reflection questions that you'll find at the end of each chapter—will be integral to this section, as you'll develop a comprehensive understanding of your strengths and impediments on the way to awakened sleep, which you can then apply in Part 3.

The goal is to provide you with a detailed framework for understanding *your* sleep. In these pages, we'll share how the quality of conscious awareness that's such a crucial component of awakened sleep can help you address emotional unhappiness, cognitive impairment, physical ailments, and spiritual well-being in a holistic way. As you read, you'll be inspired to make small changes that will have major effects, whether you're awake or asleep. You could say that all paths ultimately lead to the same mountaintop, but each individual path is paved with unique stones representing your experience in this world. Thus, although many will argue there's only a narrow set of practices you need to apply to enhance and improve your sleep, we believe the journey to awakened sleep is meant to be a reflection of each singular path. There's no one-size-fits-all panacea, but our hope is that everything you learn throughout this book will empower you to cultivate your own map that leads to the illustrious destination of awakened sleep.

MASTER YOUR SLEEP

There's an untapped potential within you, one that can be awakened by using the practices in this book. It's always been there, whether you feel it or not. With *Awakened Sleep*, you'll start to make empowered choices that work for *you*. No matter what might be getting in the way of your sleep, we want you to know that awakened sleep *is* within reach.

It's important to note that *Awakened Sleep* is not an in-depth discussion of medical sleep disorders; it is, first and foremost, a guide, informed by thousands of years of Ayurvedic and Vedic wisdom, to help you access your unique potential. At the same time, our book goes into some of the current understandings in sleep science, which is vast and evolving by the minute. While this information can be helpful, most researchers acknowledge that when it comes to sleep science, there are more questions than answers, and some aspects of sleep remain a mystery. As we strive to explain the phenomenon we call sleep, we realize that there's much more to figure out, at least from a scientific perspective.

Sleep is a subjective experience that science has tried hard to quantify and objectify. While continuing the search for objective information, we must consider and explore the *qualitative* aspects of sleep. After all, sleep is an experience, not a measurement! Every night offers a brand-new experience, based on the impact of everything you've encountered throughout the day. What your mind has absorbed and become in your waking hours is what you'll experience during sleep. You can utilize the experience of awakened sleep to process and transcend those experiences, to achieve better health and well-being.

Often, testing and a medical workup are necessary to get further information with respect to why you may be having trouble sleeping, and we encourage you to pursue workups as needed. Not being evaluated using modern tools would be like not using current technologies to test for diabetes or heart disease—and many sleep disorders have modern treatments that can and should be considered. However, as is often the case in medicine, a diagnosis is made and the solution is to treat the symptoms, not the root cause or the factors that may have created the sleep disorder in the first place. Many treatments can have long-term effects, some of which we aren't even aware of yet. Even so, we still value the perspective that modern science has to offer and encourage you to contact your physician if you are experiencing sleep challenges and to develop a deeper understanding on your own of the factors involved in your individual situation. They do not have to be mutually exclusive.

The information in *Awakened Sleep* is meant to be a valuable complement to any medical interventions. It is also for you if you have a diagnosed sleep disorder and feel you have something inherently wrong with you that you can't change. We hope *Awakened Sleep* will transform those feelings and reconnect you to your capacity for self-regulation, including the ability to sleep, that all of us are born with. We are all built to thrive, and we'll teach you how you can apply this to your sleep. Even if you take just a few of the pointers in this book to heart and experience awakened sleep for a brief period of time, you'll wake up feeling refreshed and ready to tackle the day with more awareness and purpose.

The practices in this book come from our work, which we have applied for many decades, solving the sleep problems of thousands of individuals. Maintaining regular practices to address your full body/mind/spirit wellness, you'll not only sleep better but also experience greater vitality and well-being throughout your day.

The practices of *Awakened Sleep* center on six main principles culled from Ayurvedic wisdom:

- **Stress management and meditation:** We can't avoid stress, but we can learn to manage it more effectively. We emphasize meditation and mindful awareness as a crucial way to mitigate our stressors. Awakened sleep is an extension of meditation that heals the effects of stress.

- **Emotional regulation:** Science is becoming more aware of the intimate connection between mind and body, and of emotional states as a key driver of our physiology. In Ayurveda, it's believed that the majority of physical ailments have an emotional root cause. Understanding and managing our emotions, rather than allowing our emotions to control us, is essential to our health and our sleep.

- **Nutrition:** When the body is balanced, the mind feels better. Ayurveda notes that foods can directly affect our emotional state, and science is discovering that certain nutrients are necessary for generating neurotransmitters that can influence our moods and induce sleep. We'll discuss food and nutrition as it pertains to a healthy sleep regimen.

- **Movement:** In Ayurveda, it's said that movement is life. The ancient Ayurvedic physician Sushruta was the first documented person to have prescribed regular movement for health. In this book, we discuss how movement not only assists our health during the day but also can be used in service of awakened sleep.

- **Self-care:** Self-care is especially important in setting up a daily routine, known as *dinacharya* in Ayurveda. Ayurveda recognizes the importance of not only *what* we do throughout the day but *when* we do it. Sleep researchers also understand the importance of our circadian rhythm and aligning our internal rhythms with nature's cycles for proper sleep. Ayurvedic self-care practices help us align with our natural rhythms. We'll offer several options for creating a healthy routine that promotes high-quality sleep and can be customized to your lifestyle.

- **Sleep:** Ayurveda has always recognized sleep as a biological necessity that's foundational to life. Throughout our book, we'll delve into the importance of good sleep hygiene in the hours before bed, but we expand the concept of sleep hygiene to include your activity during the day. We'll introduce you to Ayurvedic descriptions of sleep and areas of sleep that are still not well understood in modern science.

Aside from the immediate health benefits you'll experience by putting our tools into practice, you'll receive a bold (re)introduction to universal spiritual laws that'll help you unlock the keys to higher consciousness within the sleep state. With awakened sleep, you won't simply reach a neutral place; you'll tap into your greatest ability to thrive in body, mind, and spirit. You'll appreciate why a good day—and a good life—always begins the night before.

UPGRADE YOUR SOFTWARE

While you might have initially picked up this book seeking tips for a better night's sleep, the true purpose of *Awakened Sleep* is to help you catalyze higher states of consciousness. Sleep is viewed as the elixir of youth, but even more than that, it can be the gateway to awakening our spiritual intelligence.

A growing body of scientific studies suggests that human consciousness is nonlocal; that is, it's not limited to our brains, bodies, and the ways we think of space and time. Ayurveda and Vedic science have always known that consciousness and deep spiritual experience bring us into unity with all that exists. As we tap into the secrets of consciousness through sleep, we have the opportunity to access health, well-being, and creativity beyond our wildest dreams. Through the capacity to watch ourselves as we dream and sleep, we can enter the witness/observer role that helps us move beyond our limited ideas of who we are. We can come to identify not with our everyday roles and personalities, or our physical body or thoughts and emotions, but as the ocean of bliss and pure potential that is consciousness.

Over the years, we've taught thousands of people that the ingrained genetic tendencies we're born with are analogous to computer hardware, which we can't fundamentally change. However, we can upgrade our software, or our mental patterns and levels of consciousness. This book will help you understand your hardware and give you the tools to change and upgrade your software.

We teach meditation because it has the power to clear and transform our conditioned patterns and habits. In spiritual terms, it helps us disentangle from our past actions and become conscious of the thoughts, emotions, and activities that usually play out on autopilot. Science has already confirmed meditation's many health benefits, as well as its regulatory effect on sleep, and how it can harmonize the relationship between body and mind.

While meditation helps us hone our awareness in our waking hours, awakened sleep does something similar during our sleeping hours. In our view, sleep is an extension of meditation that can aid you in learning to identify with the part of the self that transcends the body, mind, thoughts, and any fixed sense of identity. Your spiritual activities (including sleep, when done with mindfulness) can optimize everything from the quality of your dreams to your overall health.

You deserve to access the peace, ease, joy, and radiance that should be part of your experience as a human being. Through this accessible course in time-honored Vedic and Ayurvedic principles, combined with the many ways Western science is validating Eastern wisdom, we're equipping you with all you need to develop a set of habits and practices that work for you.

Our invitation to you is to embark on the lifelong adventure of awakened sleep and access an awareness of your unlimited self. We're not seeking perfection over sustainability. We promise you'll find that even a few small shifts in your behavior and approach will open your eyes to the power of awakened sleep. This isn't solely about getting a few uninterrupted hours to snooze (as desirable as that might be for many of us!); it's about reentering the womb of consciousness and emerging in a place of powerful possibilities.

PART 1

THE THREE PILLARS OF WELL-BEING—HOW THEY SHAPE YOUR SLEEP AND HEALTH

CHAPTER 1

☽ ☽ ● ☾ ☾

WHAT IS AWAKENED
SLEEP?

Each night, when I go to sleep, I die. And the
next morning, when I wake up, I'm reborn.

—Mahatma Gandhi

I MAGINE THIS: YOU AUTOMATICALLY WAKE UP AT 6 A.M., WITHOUT the help of a jarring alarm, to the melody of birds outside your window and the gentle morning light flowing into your room. You feel refreshed. Your thoughts are clear. A sense of ease and vitality fills your body, and your mind is calm and alert. Rather than fussing over your to-do list, you trust that what needs to get done will get done, and you're excited for the opportunity to be present throughout it all. You're looking forward to everything the day will bring, but you're not in a rush. You take a moment to stretch before getting out of bed to do some deep breathing, intention-setting, and a meditation that'll help you remain in a state of wakeful awareness all day. After fifteen minutes, you rouse yourself further with twenty minutes of physical movement. Then, you prepare a light breakfast, which you sit down to savor at your kitchen table—sans your smartphone.

After getting ready, it's time for your morning commute, an opportunity to contemplate the beauty of the day or listen to that podcast you've been meaning to tune in to. If you work from home, you turn to your phone or computer for the first time since last night to shoot off some emails and continue a project you're eager to give your full attention to for the next few hours.

You feel relaxed yet alert, calm yet energized. Every conversation, even the ones that may bring up differing opinions or outright conflict, offers an opportunity for creative solutions. You approach all issues with a positive attitude. Others take notice of how you seem to get so much done without an enormous amount of exertion. One of your colleagues marvels at your sustained energy; you don't need that post-lunch energy boost in the form of a coffee or Red Bull. (Truth be told, you're happy with a single cup in the morning, and you appreciate it more for the taste than the stimulating effects!)

By the time your workday is over, you've experienced a sense of ease and fulfillment in both your professional and personal relationships. You don't feel exhausted, but you're happily spent from a day of activity. You take time to release the day with a breathing and meditation practice and ensure that you're able to sit down to eat a healthy meal in the early evening—something your digestive system will thank you for! You have more than enough time for leisure—catching up with family or friends while also taking time to relax from the day or attend to a few necessary chores.

By 10 p.m., you're back in bed and ready to wind down. You sink into comfort: no screens, no distracting noises, no glaring lights, no extreme temperatures. You finished your last meal about three hours ago, and you're free of the mind-altering effects of drugs, alcohol, and supplements that could influence your sleep.

Now is the time to go inward. You do some light journaling, letting go of the day and setting intentions for the next several hours of sleep, which you view as an opportunity to drift into the ocean of consciousness, so you can wake up feeling refreshed and present.

As you close your eyes and follow your breath, you're eager to ride the wave of calmness into a rejuvenating sleep. Your final thoughts reverberate with gratitude, peace, and love. After all, you recognize that these transitional states between sleeping and waking (whether emerging from sleep in the morning or tucking in at the end of the day) are pivotal moments in which to practice awareness and enhance clarity. It's easy for you to move into the sacred quietude of sleep and to wake up in the morning feeling refreshed. You understand that whatever you do throughout the day affects the way you end up going to bed, so you ensure that you're caring for your body, mind, and spirit in every waking moment.

In short, you understand and experience **awakened sleep**.

If what we've just described resonates with you, wonderful! You're fortunate to intimately know the gifts of awakened sleep, which can carry you through the day and night and into higher states of consciousness.

And if this doesn't sound like your typical routine, not to worry: Everything you're about to encounter here will help bring you back into a state of balance, which is your deepest nature (even if it may not currently feel like it), so that you can get to the blissful state of awakened sleep.

Our experiences of sleep vary according to our circumstances and context, but the following scenario might sound familiar to you, and possibly, it's more aligned with your general experience of sleep than is the first scenario.

You wake up abruptly after repeatedly hitting the snooze button on your alarm clock. You feel groggy and irritated. You may be recovering from a series of disturbing vivid dreams, or hours of tossing and turning because of your partner's snoring or street noise that was impossible to block out.

You're cranky because you're running late for work. Not to mention, your neck hurts because you were sleeping in an uncomfortable position. On top of that, your stomach feels queasy and your mind somewhat foggy because you're reeling from the effects of one too many glasses of wine at a postwork happy hour. You sigh as you think about all the work that's on your plate and all the things that haven't been crossed off your to-do list. You also notice that the TV is still on at a low drone because you fell asleep after a couple hours of binge-watching a show on Netflix (you find it hard to drift off without *some* kind of distraction in the background). You immediately recognize that you didn't get a good night's sleep (whatever that is, as it's been so long since you experienced it). You were way too stressed to doze off easily as you ruminated over a hundred different topics: work, relationships, money, and the other preoccupations that crowd your thoughts most of the time.

You groan as you rush to get ready and force yourself out the door without stopping to eat a proper breakfast. "I'll grab something at Starbucks," you say to yourself as you anxiously brace for a busy commute and a busy workday. You make a mental note to get to sleep earlier tonight, although you have the sinking sensation that even if you try, you won't shut your eyes right away. You'll be stalked by the relentless soundtrack of your monkey mind, which you've more or less gotten used to.

Unfortunately, the experience we've just described is the more common scenario. Most of us understand that awakened sleep, whose causes and effects we described in the first few paragraphs of this chapter, is an ideal state. Most of us also innately understand that beyond getting the requisite hours of sleep for our body's systems to properly function, there are other benefits—the kind that can push us out of what we consider normal. We get that sleep has a massive impact on us: physically, mentally, emotionally, and spiritually. Yet we have no idea how to change our lifestyles so that we can have the blissful experience of awakened sleep. Perhaps we've been told there's something clinically wrong with us, which we need medications to fix. We feel lost about how to even begin to improve our sleep.

If you're one of the fifty to seventy million people who struggle with sleep issues—or if you're someone whose sleep is "fine," but you're curious as to what your life might look like if you were to open the door to awakened sleep—these practices can change your life. Even if it seems like awakened sleep is out of reach—whether you're a new parent, a woman going through menopause, someone who's periodically struggled with insomnia, or someone who's dealt with the ever-increasing challenges of urban noise and light pollution—we're here to remind you that it's part of your natural state . . . a state you can be reattuned to, with some care and willingness. We will help you identify the factors contributing to the lack of awakened sleep, and what to do to experience it on a regular basis.

Awakened sleep expands our consciousness so that even when our eyes are shut, our creative capacity and ability to manifest our dreams and goals only continue to strengthen in our waking lives. As you've already seen, this can result in being clear and wide-awake in the morning, ready to face the day and whatever challenges and rewards it may bring. Awakened sleep helps us to clarify our intentions and move through perceived obstacles so that we can be a clear channel for better health and wellness.

With awakened sleep, we tap into our ability to self-regulate in both body and mind. Our internal self-regulatory mechanisms are always trying to point us toward health in the body and happiness in the mind. And although, from an Ayurvedic perspective, health and happiness are our natural state, so many circumstances and choices we make in our hectic, rapid-fire modern lives can get in the way of experiencing our underlying state of wellness. Often, we might be doing things that, unbeknownst to us, interfere with our natural sleep patterns or deprive our bodies and minds of the nutrients and care they need to induce easy, restful sleep.

This is where the traditional healing system known as Ayurveda can be a powerful guide for your overall health and wellness. *Ayurveda* is one of the world's oldest medical systems. We often refer to Ayurveda as the original lifestyle medicine, as it teaches us how to tap into our inner ability to create health on a daily basis. Its first mention was in the *Atharva Veda*, one of the four major texts of the Vedas, which are the most revered wisdom treatises of the Indian subcontinent's ancient culture.

The *Atharva Veda* was most likely set to text sometime between 1200 and 1000 BCE, and it includes a number of Ayurvedic prescriptions, as well as detailed breakdowns of anatomy and surgery—not to mention, a treasury of ideas about the metaphysical elements of Ayurvedic healing. And although it originated thousands of years ago in India, the practical tools of Ayurveda are still relevant today and apply anywhere on the planet, as they are based on the laws of nature, including human nature, which hasn't changed over time. In fact, many of the Ayurvedic concepts you'll learn will sound familiar, as most healing traditions around the world observed the same natural laws and described how to apply them to our health and well-being.

Throughout this book, we'll do our best to take some ancient concepts and customize them to fit your twenty-first-century context. If you remain curious and open, this book will empower you to move toward the kind of healthy lifestyle changes that will trigger a state of continual well-being. At first, it'll require more steadfastness and conscious awareness than usual—but as many of our patients discover, the process is far easier and more pleasurable than we think it will be at first.

THE ESSENCE OF WELL-BEING

To understand the foundations of awakened sleep, you have to understand well-being. We define **well-being as a natural state of balance in the body, mind/emotions, and spirit**. We can't have well-being without recognizing all three of these important aspects. According to Ayurveda and other forms of holistic medicine, these three areas of well-being are intertwined, and each influences the other. When we cultivate well-being in all aspects of life, we can begin the journey toward awakened sleep. Sometimes, our patients are surprised when we ask questions about many different areas of their lives and give them practices that address physical, mental/emotional, and spiritual well-being.

Physical health is what enables you to have a joyful, energetic body. The critical aspects of physical health include strong and healthy digestion and appetite, regular and effortless elimination, the capacity to fall asleep easily and sleep soundly at night, the experience of a body that's free from physical pain, and the energy and stamina to accomplish your goals on a daily basis.

Mental/emotional health refers to a reflective and alert mind that allows you to feel stable and calm in your thoughts and capable of regulating your emotions rather than feeling like you're at their mercy. You're able to view your experiences with clear eyes and find opportunities for joy and success, and you generally feel happy and hopeful, even in the midst of challenges. You accept things exactly as they are and don't struggle against what is.

Spiritual health entails a loving and compassionate heart and a lightness of being. With optimal spiritual health, you feel that your life has meaning. You experience a palpable sense of purpose that allows you to use your natural gifts and talents to serve your higher self and others. You feel a sense of connection to all beings, the planet, and something bigger than your individual self. You're easily able to spot beauty all around you and are filled with a sense of wonder and awe.

All of these elements are foundational when it comes to true well-being. Unfortunately, if we look at the world as it is, we don't have a collective sense of well-being. Heart disease, stroke, cancer, diabetes, and lung disease are responsible for 74 percent of deaths worldwide, and these noncommunicable diseases are on the rise globally.[1] One in three adults around the world has more than one chronic condition.[2] People are being diagnosed with these diseases at much younger ages than in the past. We also know that chronic pain is an epidemic worldwide. Clearly, we've missed the mark when it comes to global physical well-being.

As far as mental health, according to current mental health statistics from the World Health Organization, depression is the number one disability in the world,[3] and many health care professionals have spoken of our current global circumstances in the wake of COVID-19 as pointing to a troublesome crisis in mental health among all age, racial/ethnic, and socioeconomic groups. Mental health disorders, such as anxiety, are becoming more widespread, affecting people at younger and younger ages.

Despite many around the globe reporting that spiritual health is extremely important to them, a 2023 McKinsey Health Institute survey of employees in thirty countries revealed that spiritual well-being scores were lower relative to other measures of well-being.[4] In the modern work environment, people are having more difficulty finding meaning and purpose. As we face the realities of climate change, it's also clear that the majority of us are not experiencing a meaningful enough connection to the planet and one another.

It's no wonder people aren't experiencing awakened sleep when overall health is so compromised. And as much as our practices to create health can result in better sleep, addressing sleep itself will in turn improve our well-being. Remarkably, sleep can be a fantastic tool for helping us move toward total well-being and addressing the current deficit we seem to be experiencing among all three pillars of well-being.

To ensure that we're cultivating optimal well-being, in addition to the hours we are in bed, we must also pay attention to our choices throughout the day, including the ways we're moving and eating. By setting up a proper sleep-hygiene protocol that begins from the moment we wake up in the morning, we're empowered to take conscious responsibility for all the decisions we're making—whether we choose to hit the snooze button for twenty extra minutes or use that time to set meaningful intentions for the day ahead.

Awakened sleep can give us enough clarity to recognize all the choice points that occur throughout every moment of our day that can lead to better or worse health outcomes.

Nurture the Body: The Path to Physical Well-Being

Let's take a look at how you can prepare for awakened sleep by attending to your physical health throughout the day. Although it'll vary by individual, there are some general principles that will apply to everyone.

We recommend a whole-food, plant-based diet full of organic fruits, vegetables, nuts and seeds, healthy grains, and healthy proteins and fats to promote better sleep—which reduces inflammation in the body. A 2024 review published in *The British Medical Journal* found that eating ultra-processed food resulted in an increased risk of more than thirty health conditions, many of which play a role in sleep disruption.[5] Conversely, a Mediterranean-style diet has been repeatedly reported to reduce the risk of chronic diseases, likely due to the predominance of plant-based, anti-inflammatory foods in this diet, and to aid in better sleep.[6] In addition, the overnight fasting period has been associated with better brain health, while natural herbal teas, which contain plant-based nutrients (phytonutrients) and flavonoids (specific molecules in plants that have health benefits), can induce sleep through their sedative effects. For example, chamomile tea, which supports natural sleep, contains a flavonoid called apigenin that binds to receptors in the brain to induce sleepiness—some of these receptors are also the targets of sleep medications.

It's crucial to adopt a diet with a wide variety of nutrients, many of which can improve the quality of sleep and allow the body to function properly during the day. A 2020 review of studies looking at the effect of diet on sleep showed that dietary intake can affect sleep outcomes.[7]

Some dietary factors that were found to support sleep included a high-carbohydrate diet (whole grains), foods containing tryptophan (nuts/seeds, turkey/chicken, eggs, leafy greens) and melatonin (nuts/seeds, fish, rice, oats), and foods with specific phytonutrients, such as those in cherries and goji berries. Lower levels of certain minerals (such as magnesium and zinc) in the body can increase the risk of sleep disorders, supporting the idea that eating a wide variety of healthy foods helps reduce sleep issues.

Exercise can also be effective for better sleep. Not only does adequate physical activity during the day create a healthy exhaustion in the body, but moderate exercise also has anti-inflammatory effects.[8] Moderate physical activity is usually defined as movement that increases your heart rate and makes you sweat but allows you to talk without gasping for breath. Most people also recognize less pain, and therefore better sleep, when they are getting regular, moderate movement. The regularity of physical activity can reduce inflammation over time and set you up for restful sleep, so it's better to do some physical activity regularly than doing it in bursts. The current recommendation is getting about 150 minutes of moderate physical activity in a week. You can also practice gentle yoga poses in the evening, such as knee to chest, supine twist, forward bend, child's pose, cat/cow, and belly breathing in corpse pose to increase flexibility. You can look these poses up online or refer to our website, www.awakenedsleep.net, for some gentle yoga routines. Alternatively, when we overdo exercise (yes, there is such a thing as overexercising), we create inflammation and overstimulation that can interfere with sleep.

In fact, thousands of years ago, the Ayurvedic physician Sushruta recognized the importance of exercise for immune health and prevention of disease and defined it as a sense of weariness from bodily labor that should be done every day. He instructed patients to engage in moderate exercise (he was opposed to excessive exercise, noting that it could cause disease and even death) and took into account the age, strength, physique, and diet of the individual, as well as the season of the year and the terrain of the area, thus applying a highly personalized approach to exercise.

Keeping your physical body in balance with exercise and creating a sense of tiredness in the body can work wonders when it comes to improving your sleep patterns.

Cultivate Inner Harmony: Mental and Emotional Well-Being

In general, mental health refers to the ability to think clearly and perform cognitive functions, while emotional well-being refers to how we manage our feelings and emotions, although these terms are sometimes used interchangeably. These factors are both considered in an Ayurvedic view of the mind, which describes practices that balance both aspects.

A rested and clear mind allows you to think through situations, make decisions, and even access your intuition and creativity. When it's not cared for properly, the mind can become consumed by stress and dys-regulated emotions that can wreak havoc on health and negatively affect sleep.

You are not alone if you find that thoughts race endlessly through your mind as you try to fall asleep. This can be the result of holding on to the stress of the day, worrying about the next day, or having a general sense of anxiety that affects your ability to settle the mind. You may be ruminating on the past, replaying the day over and over in your head, or worrying about the future. In today's chronically connected world, all of us experience a high level of stimuli throughout the day and into the night. From an Ayurvedic perspective, the senses are the gateways to the mind, and all sensory input needs to be processed by the mind. Overstimulation of any of the senses, be it noisy environments or star-ing at screens all day, can create a mental state that makes it challeng-ing to fall or stay asleep.

There are several practices throughout this book to help you calm your mind and cultivate present-moment awareness. Practices such as journaling can influence the activity of various areas of the brain and help reduce feelings of stress. Journaling helps us process our emotions and cultivate a calmer and more reflective mind, which is conducive to good sleep. Researchers have shown that putting feelings into words through journaling can reduce activity in the amygdala, the part of the brain associated with stress, and activate the prefrontal cortex, the part of the brain that helps us process and regulate emotions.[9]

Meditation and breathwork are also important practices for reducing stress and calming the nervous system before bed. Yoga philosophy teaches that the breath and mind are intimately connected, and when we slow the breath, we also slow the mind. In fact, studies have shown that practicing slow, rhythmic breathing can reduce symptoms of anxiety and improve psychological well-being by modulating both the nervous system and brain activity.[10]

To cultivate a mind that is ready for awakened sleep, you can begin to remove anything that might be causing your mind to stay "turned on." Turn off any distractions at least one hour before heading to bed, which will allow your mind time to process the sensory input that has come in throughout the day. This includes disconnecting from your TV, computer, and phone (and if it's difficult to turn off your phone, at least turn on Do Not Disturb). If desired, reading an uplifting book or listening to a positive podcast prior to sleep will help bring in nourishing thoughts that you can carry into your slumbering hours.

Connect with the Divine: The Journey to Spiritual Well-Being

Connecting to your spirit is the key to awakened sleep. Your spirit is distinct from your mind, which is based on your mental processes, as well as the roles and identities you take on in your daily life. Your mind gives you a mental picture of who you are, which is based on your sense organs and the cognitive processes of the brain (including things like memories, learned behavior, etc.). In contrast, your spirit (which you might refer to as the soul, consciousness, or awareness) is outside of space and time, and its functions extend beyond the brain. It is the field of awareness within which all your physical and mental experiences are happening. It is the true, unchanging, and permanent "you" that is having this human experience. As opposed to the constantly changing experience that we call a body and mind, your spirit is the timeless and eternal you that is the source of infinite possibilities, including awakened sleep.

When you connect to your spirit, you're awakening consciousness, which gives you access to your highest potential. While mental/emotional well-being is about taking care of and regulating your thoughts and emotions, spiritual well-being helps you to recognize that there's something much greater than the separate human "I" and brings a sense of peace to life. There's an eternal source of wisdom that guides your sense of purpose throughout your daily undertakings and is the source of your inner healing ability. Your spiritual well-being can be what determines your overall health and happiness and the way you make meaning of your life, which has a huge impact on the other two pillars of well-being.

Unsurprisingly, a spirit that feels disconnected from the whole has the power to disrupt your sleep rhythms. To access your ability for awakened sleep, spiritual practices are perhaps the most important to incorporate into your life. These can include meditation, yoga, prayer, and connecting to nature. By connecting to spirit, you can create a life of meaning and purpose, which will help you become more content and less stressed. You can further develop a strong sense of spiritual well-being by connecting to something beyond your individual self, such as a community or support group, volunteer organization, friends, or family. You can also connect to your spirit by bringing your awareness to gratitude, forgiveness, empathy, and loving kindness, as many meditation practices do.

Throughout this book, you'll find suggestions for simple reflective activities, as well as more advanced practices, that will increase your capacity for awakened sleep by balancing body and mind, and connecting to spirit.

An Evening Ritual for Optimal Well-Being

Here's a quick journaling practice that can help calm the amygdala—the almond-shaped bundle of gray matter in each cerebral hemisphere that regulates how we experience our emotions. It's responsible for how we process and respond to stimuli in our environment as either danger or safety. This practice can help you quiet the mind and release the contents of your day rather than taking them into the night—and it only takes three to four minutes per night. If you make it a regular practice, you'll metaphorically remove the weeds that are cluttering the mind, plant seeds of intention, and water the soil of your life with gratitude to facilitate awakened sleep.

1. **Pick the weeds.** Begin by dumping any thoughts, issues, or concerns of the day. Just notice any thoughts that are circulating in the mind and write them down without analysis or judgment. Get them out of your head and onto a piece of paper. Think of it as releasing the energy of thoughts in the mind, thus creating space for new thoughts of your conscious choice. You can also try *recapitulation*, or going back over the events of your day without evaluation or judgment. Write down what happened in your day as objectively as possible. When you notice you had a strong feeling or emotion during the day, just label that feeling as you observe yourself, and keep going. By labeling the emotion, the part of your brain that registers stress will become less active and allow you to have more restful sleep. This should take

you less than two minutes to complete, as you are not attaching to any particular event or thought.

2. **Plant the seeds.** Now that you have picked the weeds, list three intentions or desires, or positive, present-moment affirmations in the space that you've created. They'll be seeds you plant in the field of pure consciousness, something we'll talk about a lot more in Part 2, and will blossom in time. Here are some examples. (Be specific about what applies to you in any particular moment.)
   · I let go of any guilt, resentment, or anger that I'm holding on to.
   · I am bringing in greater self-love and self-acceptance.
   · I intend to make more conscious choices with my food.
   · I am perfect the way I am.
   · I accept things as they are.
   · The universe supports me wholeheartedly and unconditionally.

You can plant new seeds every night by writing down any three intentions, desires, or affirmations. This practice will help you create new patterns of thinking and behavior in alignment with your soul's desires, as opposed to old messaging. This is the important and empowering act of rewiring your brain.

3. **Water the garden.** Now, it's time to nourish your garden with gratitude. Simply list three things you are grateful for. You can be general or specific. Here are some examples:
   · I'm grateful for the sunshine.
   · I'm grateful for my supportive friends and family.
   · I'm grateful for the nourishing food I ate today.

The *feeling* of gratitude is more important than the specifics. When we express gratitude, we are activating the more evolved part of the brain (the neocortex) that allows us to feel love, compassion, and joy and to experience emotional insight and self-regulation. In addition, our intentions manifest more easily. Over time, we begin to make choices and have evolutionary experiences that bring us greater peace.

After journaling, lie down and do some deep breathing as you transition into restful sleep.

SLEEP LIKE A SAGE WITH AYURVEDA

There are some commonalities between our modern understanding of sleep and the ancient descriptions of sleep. Ayurveda recognizes that sleep is a natural and basic impulse that is essential to all living beings, a fact that modern science is now validating. And although modern science can describe *what* happens when we sleep (and don't sleep) and has shown the importance of healthy sleep, it doesn't address the *why*. As a consciousness-based healing system, Ayurveda recognizes that sleep helps us connect to the realm of spirit, and the outcome of this is a healthy body and mind. When we experience awakened sleep and access consciousness, the source of all healing, what we create is health and happiness. In addition, Ayurveda describes the uniqueness of each individual, including their sleep patterns and tendencies, and gives us unique insights and tools.

In Ayurvedic theory, there are three types of psychophysiological principles, known as *doshas*, that determine not only our individual body/mind constitution but also the kind of sleep we might experience. We are all born with a particular proportion of these principles, or doshas. Our dominant dosha predicts the tendencies we have in all aspects of our lives, from our emotional responses to stress, to the physiological imbalances we may be susceptible to, much as our genes predict our tendencies. Our dominant dosha can even predict our sleep tendencies. And although we all have a dominant nature, or dosha, all three doshas are present in every individual and are responsible for the physiological functions in every person. These functions are influenced by our daily behaviors and lifestyle, just as we have now learned that our genes are influenced by our lifestyle, so an Ayurvedic lifestyle focuses on keeping all the doshas balanced.

To understand the doshas, we must realize that each term represents a pattern of human behavior, or a pattern of nature. They are descriptions of qualities that exist within an individual and are based on five elements that are metaphors for natural principles. These five elements are the building blocks of our lived experience. The elements of space, air, fire, water, and earth represent aspects that exist in nature and in us. A combination of these elements creates a pattern of psychophysiology. For example, space represents potential, air represents movement, fire represents transformation, water represents cohesion, and earth represents structure. Each individual comes into the world with a certain proportion of all five of these elements and their respective qualities (like a recipe with all five ingredients), but their dominant elements create their unique tendencies, including their sleep tendencies.

The three doshas are *Vata* (with a dominance of air and space), *Pitta* (fire and water), and *Kapha* (water and earth). The qualities associated with Vata are cold, light, mobile, and dry (as space and air would be described); Pitta is hot, mobile, oily, and intense (as are fire and water). Kapha's dominant qualities are cold, slow, moist, and heavy (like water and earth). Kapha is the dosha that's most closely associated with inducing sleep, as it brings about the heavy feeling that activates sleep. An excess of Kapha qualities, however, makes it challenging to wake up. In our modern society, it is easy for the qualities of Vata or Pitta to accumulate in any of us (fast-moving, intense activity, ungrounded, etc.), which can disrupt sleep. When any of the qualities of a dosha are increased for various reasons, we become imbalanced in some aspect of our physiology.

Three Doshas | Mind–Body Constitutions

VATA	PITTA	KAPHA
Movement	Transformation	Structure

| SPACE | AIR | FIRE | WATER | WATER | EARTH |

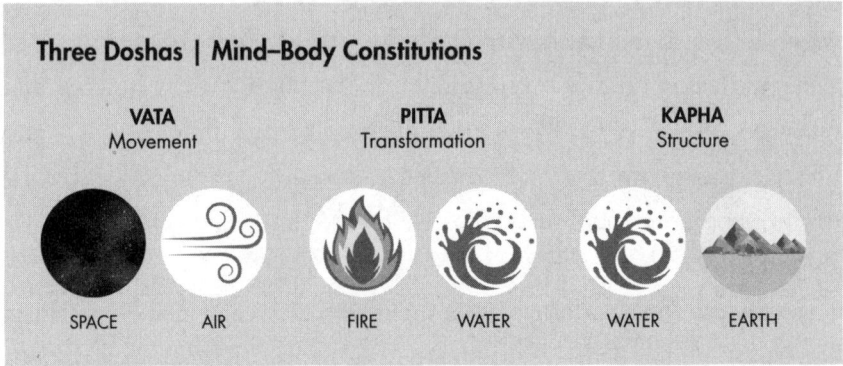

In Ayurveda, we attempt to keep all the doshas balanced, which will give us the most balanced and restorative sleep.

There is ongoing research to correlate observable dosha patterns with genes. This is the growing field known as Ayurgenomics. What we see acting out in our physiology and psychology is tied to our genes and gene expression (i.e., which genes are being actively expressed), so it makes sense that certain genetic tendencies would predict our expressed psycho-physiology. What is encoded in our genes, and how the genes are turned on or off, is ultimately what we experience.

Recent discoveries indicate that there are dozens of genes that are involved in the regulation of sleep;[11] they play a role in our natural tendencies, and genetic mutations can also predict our sensitivity to sleep deprivation. Although there is an active search for genetic treatments for sleep disruption, due to the dynamic interplay of hundreds of genes, we will not likely find a medication that can "treat" these multiple factors. Ayurveda gives us a simple way to predict sleep types, as well as tendencies toward sleep disruption, so we need only look at what is in front of us!

Ayurvedic doctors are often asked how we know certain facts about a person just by knowing their dosha. Dosha typing is a powerful tool that can help us make sense of so many of our health issues. A person's primary, or dominant, dosha can actually predict their sleep tendencies.

Many of our patients are amazed that we can predict their health tendencies and history simply by understanding their dosha.

People with a predominant Vata dosha tend to be light sleepers who also have vivid dreams. They are active and creative types. Their bodies and minds move a lot due to the qualities of space and air (movement, lightness, cold). Vata is easily overstimulated by too much activity, which is why having ample time to wind down before sleep is especially important for this type. Any activities that serve to nourish the body, mind, and spirit (like full-body massage with warm oils, which we discuss in Chapter 5) are encouraged. Grounding, slowing down, and calming the energy in the body and mind will help Vata types sleep better.

Pitta types are characterized by the qualities of fire and water (especially fire) in the body, such as heat, intensity, and acidity. They have a high degree of focus and are goal-oriented. Someone with a dominant Pitta dosha might have a hard time falling asleep if they're preoccupied with work-related stress or if they've eaten too many acidic foods. It's important for this type to eat cooling foods, reduce spicy and acidic foods (especially before bed), reduce time thinking about work and projects, and play more during the day to "cool down" and reduce their intense lifestyle. Unlike the other two doshas, Pitta people may do better with a little less sleep, making efficient use of their sleep time in the same way they do their waking hours.

Kapha types tend to be associated with calmness and stability, just like their primary elements of earth and water. Due to its slow, heavy qualities, sleep is Kapha's superpower, so they don't typically have difficulty sleeping; in fact, they can usually fall asleep anytime, anywhere. However, their quality of sleep may be compromised if they are too sluggish or inactive during the day. Exercising lightly after dinner to stimulate digestion is important for this dosha, which can struggle with low metabolism. Regular exercise reduces congestion, creates lightness, and precludes too deep a slumber. Kapha people tend to sleep heavily, which means they may be more susceptible to too much sleep or waking up groggy; thus, for a Kapha type, it's best to rise before 6–7 a.m.

Everyone has all three doshas in the body to some degree, although each of us tends to have a dominant one or two. The Sanskrit term *prakruti* refers to the nature or constitution with which you were born, whereas *vikruti* refers to your current state, or the set of imbalances you might be experiencing right now. Your prakruti does not change over your lifetime (just as your genes don't change). However, your vikruti can change moment to moment (like gene expression), as it is influenced by all your experiences and choices. Ayurveda recognizes, similar to the nature/nurture theory, that although we have our natural constitution and tendencies, our experiences and choices can influence our body and mind, and even shift us away from our tendencies. In other words, we can experience imbalances in any of the doshas depending on our lifestyle.

In order for awakened sleep and optimal well-being to be present, all the doshas need to be balanced. Imbalance occurs when there is an accumulation of one of the doshas, and therefore, the qualities of that dosha. By identifying what dosha or doshas are out of balance, Ayurveda helps to correct imbalances. If imbalances aren't corrected, this will lead to symptoms (such as sleep disruption) and, ultimately, disease.

A primary principle in Ayurveda is balancing with opposites. In other words, like increases like, and opposites balance. For example, when something is too cold, we balance by adding heat; when something is too dry, we add moisture; when something is too light, we add heaviness; and so on. If you find yourself doing this in life, you're already using the Ayurvedic principle of balance!

SYNC WITH NATURE'S RHYTHMS

Another central concept in Ayurveda is that of natural rhythms. In medicine, we are just beginning to understand the importance of daily (circadian) rhythms, not only for sleep, but for overall health. For centuries,

Ayurvedic doctors have educated patients about the daily cycles of the body and how to achieve optimal health by aligning our lifestyle with nature's rhythms.

The term *chronobiology* may be relatively new to Western medicine, but it has always been an essential part of Ayurvedic medicine. The ancient texts describe how our bodies are constantly interacting with sunlight and the changing seasons. They talk about how to synchronize one's daily routine with changes in natural light. Ayurveda may be the only medical tradition that discusses how to arrange a daily routine to achieve optimal health and well-being throughout the seasons and decades of your life. In fact, Ayurveda emphasizes that all your behaviors—including diet, rest, and exercise—must work together with your internal clock, as well as nature's clock, to keep the body functioning well.

Ayurveda is also one of the only traditions to discuss body type and how this manifests in certain health problems, including problems having to do with sleep. So much health advice assumes that everybody is more or less the same in their need for sleep, exercise, and food. However, you can see that your body isn't like anyone else's. Your personality isn't like anyone else's. You have probably already learned that what works for someone else may not work for you. Ayurveda has no concept of a single diet, exercise, or sleep routine that is correct for every single person, or that is correct for a person throughout their whole life. While everyone needs to understand how to set a good general schedule, not everyone needs exactly the same sleep protocol within that schedule to get the best results.

Throughout this book, we'll describe how you can identify and resolve your particular challenges with sleep, taking into account your unique dosha constitution and what dosha may be out of balance in your life. Just as we inherently know that we are not the same day-to-day, year-to-year, decade-to-decade, our needs can also shift. In taking your own unique needs into consideration, you can set a basic sleep schedule and routine that will support your body's rhythms, and you'll also be able to fine-tune it so that sleep will become effortless and restorative at different times in your life.

According to Ayurveda, the quality of your day depends on the quality of sleep you received the night before—and the quality of your day then affects the sleep you'll get at night. It's a constant feedback loop that requires conscious attention. The type of preparation you make for awakened sleep will depend on the kind of sleeper you are. Most people think of themselves as night owls or early risers, but it's more complicated than that. You could be a light sleeper who has difficulty falling asleep or a heavy sleeper who struggles to wake up; further, some people fall asleep easily but wake in the wee hours due to stress or restlessness, and then might sleep through their alarm clock and wake up feeling groggy and dull.

The assessment at the end of the chapter will help you determine your particular style of sleep; this will inform the sleep protocol you'll be designing (which the remaining chapters will begin to help you build). Keep in mind that, as you respond to each of the questions in the assessment, you'll be basing your responses not on what might be occurring in your sleep at this point in your life (which can be influenced by lifestyle and current circumstances), but on trends you've encountered in your quality of sleep throughout your life.

Answer the questions to the best of your ability and discover how you might be able to unlock the door to awakened sleep. There will be a variety of assessments throughout the book that build on this one and help you better understand what you need in order to make your waking and sleeping life as restful, balanced, and awakened as possible.

Once you have your sleep routine in place, you'll notice an increase in your level of energy and focus, and your mood will improve. You may also notice your physical symptoms improve. Understanding your own nature is what will help you get out of a disruptive sleep pattern and open the door to awakened sleep. All it takes is a deeper understanding of yourself and your basic constitution.

HOW AWAKENED SLEEP CAN MANIFEST

We recently met a client, a forty-six-year-old executive named Marsha, who'd just gotten off sleep medication in the hopes of settling into a more natural rhythm that supported her overall well-being. Marsha lived in the San Francisco Bay Area, where she had a high-level job in the financial sector. She was going through menopause and had a difficult time falling and staying asleep. As a longtime meditator, Marsha was trying to incorporate meditation into her life on a daily basis. However, her mornings were too busy for her to devote a full twenty minutes to the practice; instead, she took two to five minutes to do some deep breathing, but the effects didn't linger over the rest of her day. She was usually tired in the morning and entered her busy and stressful job unhappy, exhausted, and in a mental fog. She found little pleasure in her work.

Marsha spent her days running around in a frenzy trying to cross things off her to-do list. She had little to no time to care for herself by exercising or eating nourishing meals. It was little wonder that she ended up feeling mentally and physically spent at the end of the day! Like many people who struggle with getting to sleep at night, the TV was her faithful evening companion that helped her numb out from frazzled or troubling thought patterns. As a single woman who'd been through a painful divorce just a few years prior, she felt lonely and frustrated, and she hadn't had time to fully work through her emotions around the relationship ending. On top of this, she habitually engaged with unhealthy beliefs that made her feel worse. She would eat something that was easy to prepare but not always healthy, and then she typically fell asleep from exhaustion in front of the TV, with a flurry of stressful and unsupportive thoughts lingering in her mind.

When she came to us for help, we assessed her overall well-being, which included looking at her lifestyle in closer detail. As she already felt overwhelmed, we focused on her evening routine first. Since mornings were challenging, we shared with Marsha that the evening could be an ideal time to incorporate a meditation and settle down after a hectic day. This ran counter to her habit of overstimulating her senses with TV when she got home. After meditating, she could make a simple meal using healthy ingredients and take time to be fully present as she ate. We recommended she remove the TV from her bedroom and instead create a soothing ritual before bed. We advised her to take a warm shower in the evening, and then massage the soles of her feet with coconut oil before she lay down in bed. We explained that in Ayurveda, the soles of the feet contain important *marma*, or acupressure, points that facilitate greater health in all our organs and tissues. According to Ayurveda, the eyes are connected to the feet, so massaging the feet can cool down heat in the eyes and reduce the impacts of staring at a screen for long periods of time—something Marsha did on a daily basis.

We told Marsha that the ideal bedtime for her was 9:30–10:00 p.m. At first, she was reluctant because she feared that she wouldn't be able to get to sleep, especially without TV to help her wind down. However, she agreed that she would try lying in bed at that time with the lights turned off, so that she could take a few minutes to think about the entirety of her day as if she were watching a film reel. She would witness the activities she'd engaged in, including things as mundane as what she'd eaten. We suggested that Marsha learn to compassionately notice her thoughts and actions without attaching judgments or emotions to them.

After recounting the day, she would engage in a deep-breathing exercise while lying flat on her back, before slowly relaxing into meditation with her palms turned up in a receptive gesture. Marsha was a practitioner of mantra meditation, so she was told to begin repeating her mantra as she drifted to sleep. While repeating the mantra, she would witness her thoughts as they came and went, not attaching to anything. This was a big shift for Marsha, who had been taught that meditation should occur only with a straight back in front of an altar. We assured her that the type of meditation we were recommending could be seen as preparation for the next seven to eight hours of her life. She could view sleep as an extension of her meditation practice that would enable her to relax her mind and body and let go of the thoughts that usually kept her up.

For the first few weeks, the practice took twenty to thirty minutes to complete. Over time, after fifteen minutes, Marsha would slowly begin to drift off. During her meditation, she would set the intention to relax her body, and as she continued to repeat her mantra, the thoughts that flitted across her mind became more vague until they melted away.

Over time, the quality of Marsha's sleep was showing clear improvement, but she was concerned that she often found herself waking at 4 a.m. She wondered if she should try to do something that would get her back to sleep. We told her that if this was her body's natural wakeup time, she should take it as a sign that the night was over and she was ready to go about her day, but Marsha was afraid that getting up at such an early hour would make her more tired during the day. We assured her that if she stayed with it, this would not be the case.

Marsha eventually developed a healthy sleep routine that worked for her. She was asleep by 10 p.m. and awake by 5:30 a.m. She used the next hour to do her morning routine, practice meditation for a full twenty minutes, eat breakfast, and get to her office by 8 a.m. By this time, she was wide-awake, with a clear and lucid mind.

Marsha told us that removing the TV from her room and connecting with a simple meditation practice that set her mind at ease had been extremely helpful. A month or two after she made all these changes, she came back to us with some exciting updates. Although she'd spent a few years feeling lonely and longing for connection, she'd recently met a wonderful man who fulfilled her need for spiritual partnership. When she first came to us, she also expressed concern over some common menopausal symptoms, including brain fog and difficulty recalling information. With her new sleep protocol, she felt a greater degree of physical vitality, mental acuity, and spiritual peace than she had in years. Her health and well-being continued to improve as she manifested even more of her intentions.

Marsha is a glowing example of how awakened sleep can influence us on multiple levels. She used her evening routine and meditation to calm her body and mind and access the field of consciousness—and the effects rippled through her life. Throughout this book, we'll share similar techniques to the ones we shared with Marsha. Each of us is different, with our own unique context and circumstances, so you will find many practices to choose from that will work best for you. We trust that you'll see aspects of your own situation in these pages, and we hope this will be a reminder that awakened sleep is possible for everyone.

ASSESSMENT: WHAT KIND OF SLEEPER ARE YOU?

This assessment will help you identify your natural sleep type based on your dominant mind/body type (dosha). Your answers should be based on your general sleep patterns throughout most of your life, not necessarily how your sleep is right now. This assessment is meant to help you understand your prakruti (natural constitution).

All answers will be in a yes/no format. Give yourself a score of 1 for all "yes" answers, and a score of 0 for all "no" answers. Because each of us contains all three doshas in varying proportions, you'll likely have a final number for each section, but pay attention to the area(s) with the highest score to determine your primary sleep type. You may have two scores that are more or less equal, which is not unusual, as many people have two dominant doshas.

Light Sleeper (Vata)

1. Do you have a hard time falling asleep?
2. Does your sleep get easily disturbed with any noise?
3. Do you often feel cold at night?
4. Is your sleep affected by your sensory experiences (for example, the TV shows you watch, what you eat or drink, the stimuli you're subjecting yourself to) before bed?
5. Is your sleep negatively affected by travel and change of location or time zone?
6. Do you often wake up early and feel that you didn't get deep enough sleep?
7. Do you have nightmares and/or vivid, multisensory dreams?
8. If you have a poor night of sleep, do you wake up feeling anxious, jittery, and spacey?
9. After a good night's sleep, do you feel particularly happy and relaxed during the day?

Score: _____

Medium Sleeper (Pitta)

1. Do you fall asleep easily but tend to wake up around 2 a.m.?
2. Do you often feel warm and sweaty in your sleep, with a tendency to kick off the covers?
3. Do you feel as if your body is relaxed, but your mind is still awake and working while asleep?
4. Do you often feel thirsty or hungry throughout the night?
5. Do you often wake up feeling wired and planning your day?
6. Is your sleep affected by lights in the bedroom?

7. Do you have intense or violent dreams?
8. If you have a poor night of sleep, do you wake up feeling cranky or irritated?
9. After a good night's sleep, do you feel particularly focused and alert during the day?

Score: _____

Deep Sleeper (Kapha)

1. Do you tend to fall asleep easily and stay asleep through the night?
2. Do you stay asleep despite noise or distractions in the room?
3. Do you tend to fall asleep watching TV or reading?
4. Do you tend to wake up congested at night or in the morning?
5. Is the quality of your sleep negatively affected by cold temperatures in your bedroom?
6. Do you typically wake up feeling groggy?
7. Do you generally have difficulty recalling your dreams or suspect that you don't dream at all?
8. If you have a poor night of sleep, do you wake up feeling heavy and sluggish?
9. After a good night's sleep, do you feel particularly energized and motivated during the day?

Score: _____

Once you've determined your score and your dominant dosha(s), you'll have valuable information that'll be pivotal in determining whether you require a Vata, Pitta, or Kapha balancing regimen.

REFLECTIONS

1. What's your general experience of sleep? In what state do you typically fall asleep? How do you typically wake up?
2. Have you cultivated any helpful nighttime rituals (whether practiced consistently or not) that make it easier to sleep?
3. Reflect on the three pillars of well-being (physical, mental/emotional, and spiritual). Which of these three aspects feels the most challenging? Which feel like areas where you may already be experiencing robustness and/or wellness? (Please don't worry if all these aspects feel "off" for you right now; the aim of this book is to increase your awareness, not your judgments!)
4. What have your experiences of forming new habits and changing old ones been like, to date?

List any takeaways from this chapter that you'd like to incorporate into your own sleep-hygiene routine:

_____

_____

_____

_____

_____

CHAPTER 2

)) ● ((

WHY AREN'T WE
SLEEPING?

A ruffled mind makes a restless pillow.

—Charlotte Brontë

YOU'RE BORN PROGRAMMED WITH THE SACRED CAPACITY FOR SLEEP. As a baby, you naturally fell asleep on your own as long as your basic needs for warmth, safety, and nourishment were sufficiently met. So, what happened? Why did you lose that intrinsic capacity to sleep like a baby? Why do so many of us grow out of this natural ability to experience the full restoration of the body, mind, and spirit that comes from a good night's sleep?

This chapter answers the question "Why aren't we sleeping?" in depth, for the purpose of helping you increase your awareness of your sleep patterns so you can determine what may not be working in your favor—and conversely, what you can do more of to naturally induce awakened sleep.

In the last chapter, we discussed a person's inherent sleep tendencies based on their primary dosha. Although there are some differences, all types have the natural capacity for awakened sleep. But for a third of the global population, something happens that causes people to struggle with sleep in some way.

Maybe you used to be able to fall asleep without any issues—you could doze off sitting on a couch in the midst of a party, or you could pop on some headphones and snooze uninterrupted all the way through a red-eye flight. But now, you toss and turn and wake up cranky, tired, and unfocused. Or maybe you're someone who always needed a little help, so you developed your own personal sleep kit, stocked with all the stuff that helped you get good, uninterrupted sleep. Memory foam? Check! Eye mask and ear plugs? All good! Curtain clips? Lights out! But now, despite these tools, you lie awake, unable to get into a restful sleep state. And it's possible that you're utterly confused about your patterns, which seem to shift at the same breakneck speed and unpredictability as social media algorithms (which, admittedly, you've been guilty of trying to figure out into the wee hours of the morning)!

Whatever the case, taking a moment to think about how *you* sleep is an important way to gain life-changing awareness. You can't improve your sleep until you know *why* you're not sleeping. And even if you feel disheartened by thinking about your sleep issues, we want you to rest assured that it's not permanent. Because no matter what your current relationship to sleep is, each of us is born with the innate capacity to do it. In most cases, our lifestyle and choices are affecting our sleep, creating imbalances in the doshas that are interfering with it, although we might not realize it.

In the upcoming pages, we'll go through a comprehensive exploration of the common factors that tend to keep us from awakened sleep. These include a myriad of possibilities, some of them glaringly obvious, although we don't always connect the dots as to how they might be influencing our sleep. In fact, in many cases, we think these things are actively helping us; while this could be true in the short term, they often end up hindering us in the long term.

Let's explore why sleep feels like such a rare commodity for so many of us. And let's start to consider ways we can shift our focus and habits through simple steps that lead to dramatic results.

WHAT'S BLOCKING YOUR SLEEP AND HOW TO FIX IT

Most sleep issues can be traced back to two interconnected causes. The first is that we've experienced a specific interference, external or internal, that's hampering our natural ability to fall and stay asleep. Something is actively getting in the way of our natural sleep mechanisms. The second is that the complex system of our body/mind/spirit is out of balance because it isn't receiving the support it needs. Unsurprisingly, interference and lack of support usually go hand in hand.

You might be wondering, *Well, how do I know what's interfering? How do I support healthy sleep?*

It begins with awareness. We're conditioned to relegate any difficulty sleeping to something unavoidable, such as stress, illness, or getting older, so that sleep troubles become par for the course. After trying a few remedies, we might move from curiosity to resignation—when we believe that nothing can be done about our sleep troubles, because, of course, we've tried all the sleep solutions, and none of them has worked so far.

How might you describe your own quality of sleep, as well as your attempts to improve it? It's possible that many of the things you've tried that didn't end up working actually contributed to ongoing cycles of sleeplessness or poor sleep. It may be that what you tried wasn't what you needed at that time to achieve balance. It's also possible that any of the things you've turned to, including self-medicating with alcohol and pharmaceuticals to help you get through the stress of the day and combat the discomfort of yet another sleepless night, end up perturbing your natural sleep cycle. You may be looking outside yourself for answers when going within with awareness will bring you the answers you need.

As we've learned throughout our work, awakened sleep isn't just about what you're doing right before bed. It's the result of going about your entire day with a focus on balance. How you sleep is a reflection of your day, which consists of the micro and macro choices you make—often in a nanosecond, without a great deal of forethought or reflection.

We've both worked with patients who insist that they've implemented all the habits they've been advised to, ranging from warm baths to lavender aromatherapy to unplugging their electronic devices—yet a good night of truly restorative sleep feels close to impossible for them. In many cases, they end up getting prescriptions for sleep medications because they just don't know what else to do!

Your habits of caring for yourself in all dimensions come to define how and whether you're sleeping well. We want to empower you with knowledge and awareness so you can begin to take your health and well-being into your own hands. Starting with uncovering the reasons you might not be getting a good night's sleep is a powerful initiation into awakened sleep.

Western science and medicine are still figuring out what the proper protocols for good sleep hygiene are, and studies can be conflicting. Of course, in medicine, the general consensus is that we *should* be working on all aspects of our physical and mental health, ranging from getting physical movement every day to undergoing cognitive behavioral therapy. All these things can be exceptionally helpful and have likely been recommended to you by your medical practitioner. However, what we're recommending (and what we've found works) is getting a sense of the deeper reasons behind *why* you might not be sleeping. Sometimes, the solution lies in the body and sometimes in the mind; other times, it requires transcending both body and mind to look at the spiritual dimension. And, in most cases, the solutions lie in all three dimensions.

Let's look at the possible imbalances that might be leading to a lack of sleep through the framework of all three pillars of wellness. For example, while many of us recognize imbalances related to the mind or body, it's possible that a lack of sleep can be tied to your experience (or lack thereof) of deeper meaning and connection to yourself in the world, which has a more spiritual basis.

Many of these imbalances come from behaviors and habits that accumulate over time. A lot of them can begin at a young age or at an important transitional period in life. Take note of how many of them could be currently interfering with your sleep.

Body
- feeling restless (from a lack of or too much movement)
- pain or discomfort (acute or chronic)
- feeling too hot or too cold (which may be related to difficulty with thermoregulation caused by a hormonal imbalance)
- digestive issues, such as gas, cramping, bloating, heartburn, and reflux (which might stem from dietary issues or the tendency to eat too close to bedtime)
- nasal congestion (which can worsen while lying down and also increase the risk of snoring)
- medical conditions (including cancer, diabetes, heart disease, and hormonal issues, all of which can be disruptive to sleep patterns)
- taking medications that can adversely affect the quality of sleep (following is a list of the most commonly prescribed medications that can directly interfere with certain aspects of sleep):
   - antidepressants: Some can be activating and disrupt sleep (such as fluoxetine and venlafaxine) while others have a sedative effect (such as doxepin, nortriptyline, and trazodone) and may lead to morning grogginess. In addition, some antidepressants can worsen or induce

sleep disorders, such as restless leg syndrome, teeth
grinding, rapid eye movement (REM) sleep disorders,
nightmares, and sleep apnea.[1]
o antianxiety medications and sedatives, such as
   benzodiazepines
o blood pressure medications, including beta-blockers and
   ACE inhibitors
o cholesterol-lowering medications
o thyroid medications
o corticosteroids
o antiseizure medications that are also used for pain
   conditions
o weight-loss drugs
o asthma medications
o over-the-counter cold medicines, especially
   decongestants
o antibiotics
o sleep medications themselves, such as orexin receptor
   antagonists and sedative hypnotics (including zolpidem)

Mind
- feeling overstimulated during the day or in the hours
  before bed
- inability to shut off the monkey mind
- replaying the events of the day
- ruminating on the past
- feeling anxious about the future
- thinking about your to-do list
- feeling generally stressed (from work or relationship
  issues)

Spirituality

- a general lack of meaning and purpose
- feelings of isolation and loneliness
- intense bereavement and grief
- numbness and lack of connection to the world around you
- generalized feelings of fear that transcend personal circumstances (e.g., existential dread about the state of the world)
- lack of connection to spiritual or soul-based teachings, especially in difficult or transitional times

You might recognize one or more of these factors that may be interfering with your sleep. Many of them are the basis of diagnoses in medicine, and others are symptoms that may be ignored because they don't fall under a particular diagnosis. As you read on, you'll gain insight into how these things affect sleep and find tools to help, regardless of the cause.

SLEEP AIDS: HELP OR HINDRANCE?

In her primary care setting, Dr. Sheila treats a range of health conditions with lifestyle and herbs (when they can be used safely and effectively) instead of medications. She often sees people who want to treat their insomnia with supplements instead of medications. Although supplements or herbs can be safer than medications, they are not totally without potential for harm and still work best in the context of a healthy and balanced lifestyle, and when used in the short term to correct the root cause.

In addition, although many herbs and supplements can be useful to create better sleep, long-term data is still needed for most. For example, melatonin is the drowsiness-causing "sleep hormone" that the brain produces in response to darkness. Many people will resort to a melatonin supplement in order to better the quality of their sleep, as it is generally considered safe. It can be an effective short-term treatment for conditions such as jet lag and shift-work disorder. Dr. Sheila has many patients who, in an attempt to treat their sleep issues naturally, become dependent on melatonin or other supplements; she often finds that they stop working when taken for more than a few months as tolerance can develop. This can lead to people taking higher and higher doses of melatonin over time while still reporting poor sleep and not feeling rested in the morning. Clearly, there are still things to be learned, but ultimately, reconnecting to our own natural release of melatonin is the best long-term solution.

Both of us work with clients who resort to stronger prescription medication. Several years ago, a patient named Justin came to Dr. Suhas because he was concerned about his habit of using sleep meds to get to sleep. Though he didn't use them every night, Justin, a surgeon, was already feeling less bright-eyed and bushy-tailed in the mornings than he was accustomed to, so although he worried about getting the requisite amount of sleep, he knew that taking a sleeping pill could make it more difficult to fall asleep the night after.

Most of our patients recognize that sleep aids can be a double-edged sword. On the one hand, it's great to drift off quickly (especially if they've had any difficulty sleeping), but on the other, they feel that it's not ideal to take a pill in order to do something that all of us should be able to do naturally.

Additionally, most of us recognize that sleep aids aren't the solution to the sleep crisis we are in. Doctors write approximately forty million prescriptions for sleep meds every year, but half of adults still complain that they can't get adequate sleep. Although sleep aids can be tempting in the few minutes before bedtime, anyone who uses them would be well supported by a deeper understanding of the effects they might have in the long term.

Many of the classes of sleep drugs can be addictive, so they're classed as controlled substances. Many of them also have a long half-life (the amount of time your body needs to metabolize a half dose), meaning your liver could still be metabolizing them after ten hours. In fact, some require close to a full day to completely exit the body. Among people ages forty-five to sixty-four, it's been shown that sleep meds are associated with a 48 percent increase in the risk of dementia.[2]

In general, the older you are, the more time your body will need to fully metabolize the drug and be free of its effects, which could include grogginess, an impaired memory, and poor coordination—ironically, the same side effects people report after not getting a good night's sleep! Therefore, it's clear that apart from putting us to sleep, these meds have other detrimental effects on our brain health. And although sleep deprivation has also been shown to increase the risk of dementia, it doesn't seem that meds are the best solution.

Another topic that bears addressing is the use of alcohol to unwind and fall asleep. It has been estimated that approximately 20 percent of people use alcohol to manage insomnia. Individuals with alcohol use disorder are at high risk of insomnia and other sleep disorders. As a central nervous system depressant, alcohol does make us tired and has been shown to reduce the amount of time it takes before the onset of sleep. However, as most people quickly realize, it's not the same quality of sleep that we get naturally. A 2022 UK study concluded that even low levels of alcohol consumption may affect sleep health, particularly by increasing the risk of snoring.[3]

In addition to alcohol, many people use cannabis products for sleep problems. However, recent reviews and meta-analyses show that there is insufficient evidence to support using cannabis for sleep disorders.[4] In fact, data collected from people who regularly use cannabis for various medical issues suggests that it can actually worsen sleep, increase night-time awakenings, and decrease total sleep duration.[5]

Again, it's crucial to have a better understanding of the potential short- and long-term effects of sleep aids, whether they are prescribed or you're self-medicating—which could also end up interfering with other medications or supplements you're simultaneously taking.

For those suffering from insomnia, the current first line of recommendation is cognitive behavioral therapy for insomnia (CBT-I), as it's been shown to produce long-lasting results for patients who suffer from insomnia.[6] This is a nonmedication, evidence-based technique that identifies thoughts and behaviors that are contributing to sleep issues and teaches people to shift the interfering behaviors or thoughts. It is best done with the guidance of a trained therapist; however, there are now various digital programs that are quite effective as well and that may be more accessible to people. Because it addresses some of the root causes of sleep issues, the benefits of CBT-I are typically long-lasting. And while more research is necessary, evidence suggests that mindfulness meditation and yoga nidra (which we'll discuss further in Chapters 7 and 8) may improve sleep quality on a level similar to exercise or CBT-I.[7] Researchers believe this improvement could have something to do with how mindfulness techniques can decrease thoughts and mental processes that disrupt sleep. (If you're interested in CBT-I, you can find more information about locating a certified therapist in the Resources section of this book.)

As we've learned throughout our medical practices, there are many routes to improved sleep. At the same time, if you're someone who uses sleep aids of some kind because you're desperate for at least a few hours of restorative shut-eye, please know that you can still experience awakened sleep. Sleep medication can be helpful for many people; we're not opposed to it, but everything needs to be selected with awareness. Many people tend to resort to medication without exploring other options, or the options are never discussed with them. And our experience as a Western physician and an Ayurvedic doctor is that meds or supplements are best used as temporary fixes until we solve the root of the issue. When we don't get to the root cause, we end up depending on external measures, which can be difficult to wean off and can actually disrupt the quality of our sleep.

Dr. Sheila saw Jessica, a twenty-eight-year-old who came in as a new patient wanting help weaning off her meds because she was having difficulty doing it on her own. She had been prescribed the meds by her previous health care provider when she was going through a stressful time and experiencing anxiety symptoms and insomnia. Jessica was immediately put on an SSRI for her anxiety and trazodone to help her sleep, which did help in the short term. She was not taught any other practices, nor did she have a conversation about how long she would need to be on the medications. The impression she was given was that it would likely be long term because she's just a "bad sleeper," and she was told it's better to sleep with meds than not at all.

Jessica tried to gradually get off the meds; her life had become less stressful, and she didn't feel she needed to be on them anymore. She was already practicing good sleep hygiene, so Dr. Sheila helped her to incorporate additional practices for anxiety and calming down the nervous system, such as deep breathing and journaling. Gradually, she weaned herself off the meds entirely, with the help of some Ayurvedic herbs (ashwagandha, tulsi, and brahmi) and close follow-up. Over a period of three months, she was able to permanently stop taking both her meds, and she maintained good sleep in the long term by continuing regular healthy practices, with only occasional use of herbs when needed.

In reality, most medications for sleep issues, if used, should be prescribed only for the short term. They are quick and easy solutions, like spraying weed killer on weeds in the garden. But tending to the soil and nourishing the garden are the best long-term solution, with minimal, if any, need for the weed killer.

Herbs and Supplements—Supporting Natural Sleep

There are a number of herbs and natural supplements that can assist in awakened sleep. Many Ayurvedic herbs can help support sleep by calming the central nervous system or by modulating the stress response in the body (adaptogens). From an Ayurvedic perspective, herbs work by balancing doshas in the physiology, thus allowing natural sleep to occur.

- **amalaki:** considered to be the fruit of immortality; balances all the doshas (especially balances Pitta); reduces inflammation and cultivates a gentle, awakened quality in the mind
- **ashwagandha:** a grounding adaptogenic herb and mild sedative that supports neuromuscular strength and balances Vata; especially effective for debilitation/exhaustion and insomnia related to anxiety and stress
- **brahmi:** supports overall brain health and the cultivation of spiritual consciousness; commonly used to treat insomnia and anxiety; in combination with other herbs, can be even more potent
- **gotu kola:** a version of brahmi that is extremely calming and reduces Pitta
- **jatamansi:** an overall rejuvenative for the mind, it's helpful for insomnia, it calms the nervous system, and it boosts memory; beneficial for all doshas
- **jyotishmati:** an overall brain tonic for all doshas, it promotes memory and learning and illuminates the mind

- **sandalwood:** has a cooling, calming quality; particularly effective at soothing Pitta imbalance
- **shankhapushpi:** commonly used to calm the nervous system and balance all doshas; relieves stress and anxiety and promotes sleep
- **tulsi (holy basil):** considered a sacred plant, it dispels sluggishness and congestion; acts as an adaptogen to relieve stress; increases awareness and spiritual clarity; especially effective for balancing Vata and Kapha doshas
- **vacha:** calms the nervous system and supports digestion; opens the mind and has a slight hallucinogenic quality; can reduce mental sluggishness; especially useful for Vata and Kapha imbalances

Many of the aforementioned Ayurvedic herbs can be used in different formats: pills, elixirs, tinctures, jams, ghee (clarified butter), etc. We recommend consulting with an Ayurvedic specialist who can guide you further, as the proper herbal treatments and duration of treatment will vary for each person.

Because of the growing interest in natural remedies for sleep issues, research is ongoing to find safe and effective treatment options. Other herbs and natural supplements that have calming effects and can be used to support sleep include the following:

- **CBD oil:** can be used to relieve chronic pain, inflammation, depression, and anxiety
- **chamomile:** aids in muscle relaxation, alleviation of anxiety, and digestive symptoms
- **glycine:** an anti-inflammatory amino acid that can improve cognitive health, enhance mood, and aid in better sleep
- **L-theanine:** can improve cognitive function, alleviate stress, and aid in sleep and relaxation
- **lavender:** can reduce pain and inflammation, enhance mood, and improve sleep

- **lemon balm:** can relieve digestive issues and alleviate depression and anxiety
- **maca:** may relieve menopausal symptoms (which can exacerbate sleep-related conditions), and improve mental health and cognitive function
- **magnesium (citrate + glycinate):** magnesium citrate can help with muscle relaxation and reducing tension, while magnesium glycinate is highly bioavailable, aiding in deeper sleep cycles and improving overall sleep quality
- **magnolia bark:** a natural sedative that can reduce stress and alleviate insomnia
- **melatonin:** best for people experiencing jet lag, for shift workers, and for elderly people; best for short-term use
- **passionflower:** can be beneficial for anxiety, restlessness, overwork, and muscle tension
- **valerian:** can improve sleep latency (the time it takes to fall asleep after turning in for bed) and quality of sleep

Before taking any of the recommended herbs or supplements, be sure to discuss with your health care provider, especially if you are concurrently taking any other medications. The best choice of herb or supplement, current dosing, and duration of therapy can vary, and ongoing monitoring is recommended. If your current provider is not knowledgeable or open to these options, we encourage you to explore other experienced practitioners who can help guide you.

INSOMNIA—IT'S NOT A DISORDER; IT'S A SYMPTOM

From a Western medical perspective, we consider insomnia to be a medical condition, but according to Ayurveda and other forms of holistic medicine, it's a symptom related to an underlying imbalance—not a disorder in and of itself. The key is to identify what is causing the underlying imbalance and remedy that. Ayurveda reveals the necessity of reconsidering how we diagnose disorders; instead of slapping a label on a series of symptoms, it's a good idea to consider the bigger picture.

A couple of years ago, Dr. Suhas met Claudia, a fifty-six-year-old corporate professional whose postpandemic workplace scenario shifted to being at home full-time. Claudia was the main breadwinner in her family and a mother of two young children. She had so much to do in the evenings that she pushed through her sleepiness to get things done for her family and for work. She found it increasingly difficult to engage in self-care, such as walking, which she had been doing before. She began noticing weight gain and nasal congestion. She also often felt lethargic, dull, and heavy throughout the day, so she sought help from her primary care doctor. He suggested she undergo a sleep study to determine whether she had sleep apnea. She was diagnosed with sleep apnea and placed on a continuous positive airway pressure (CPAP) machine. Unfortunately, it proved to be uncomfortable, and although her Apnea-Hypopnea Index (or AHI, a system of measurement that evaluates pauses in breathing, or apneas, that happen during each hour of sleep) was acceptable and the apnea was improved, she still felt horrible in the morning. That was when one of Claudia's colleagues suggested she visit Dr. Suhas.

When he evaluated her holistically, it became clear her sleep apnea was only one symptom of a larger problem. Due to the stress from the pandemic, along with changes in her already-stressful work situation, Dr. Suhas determined that Claudia had a significant Vata imbalance. Dr. Suhas also noted that this had resulted in high blood pressure and weight gain in the prior months, which are signs of a Kapha imbalance in the body. Therefore, Claudia's "prescription" included multiple shifts in her lifestyle that addressed body, mind, and spirit and the root causes of her symptoms, addressing all the dosha imbalances that were occurring.

Dr. Suhas placed Claudia on a Vata-balancing regimen that would help her feel more centered and energized. He suggested dietary regulations that would counteract the effects of her sedentary job and poor sleep. He helped her plan her meals such that her main meal was in the middle of the day, with a light dinner. To reduce the Kapha imbalance in the body, he suggested fasting after 6 p.m. and through the morning, in addition to cutting out refined flour, heavy grains, and dairy—all of which were creating excess heaviness in the body. Claudia was also given a special Ayurvedic tea blend to help her metabolism and mood. He advised her to do some brisk cardiovascular exercise in the morning, with a light walk in the evening. Claudia also learned a meditation technique that she practiced twice a day. All these methods helped Claudia to shift her nervous energy, especially as she was going to sleep—a time during which she tended to stress over work issues.

As the hub of her family's wheel, Claudia was given the emotional support, knowledge, and motivation she needed to make massive changes. After about two months, she lost fifteen pounds and was starting to feel better in the mornings. At this point, Dr. Suhas surmised that she would probably be able to go to bed without her sleep apnea machine, so she did a trial off the CPAP—and she felt great! After another month, Claudia had lost a total of twenty-one pounds and she looked and felt like a different person: vibrant, energized, and more at peace.

Claudia participated in a repeat sleep study and found that she was sleeping much better, without any congestion or blocking of her airways. Her doctors were impressed and told her to continue what she was doing. Today, Claudia is finding more joy at work and is set to retire in two years. She's excited about the chapter that lies ahead of her, knowing that she's tackled the issues that were compounding her sense of burnout and poor sleep.

The wonderful thing about Claudia's case is that it exemplifies the ways in which clinicians often focus on a single symptom and not on the whole picture. Disorders like sleep apnea are sometimes treated as though they're fixed disease states, but focusing on the root causes can resolve the issues more permanently. Rather than treating the symptom (sleep apnea, in this case), we can investigate other aspects of a patient's life that might be contributing to an imbalance. When we do this, not only is one problem addressed—several other aspects of their health and well-being are also improved.

We often see people whose life circumstances and stressors create barriers to good sleep. We worked with a fifty-six-year-old computer engineer named Anita. Anita's mother was hospitalized in India, and as her parents' only child, she constantly traveled between the US and India. Within three months, she'd made four visits—staying up to fifteen days and traversing various time zones to come home to her work and family. After those three months, her mother passed away, at which point Anita brought her father to the US for a few months so he wouldn't be alone.

The stress of this period took a huge toll on Anita's health. She tried to stay strong for her family as they dealt with their grief, which was exhausting. She felt fearful and depressed, and so did her dad. She couldn't function or focus, and her insomnia was so acute that she was unable to sleep at night. She tossed and turned and often fell asleep during the day—becoming drowsy when she was behind the wheel or after she'd eaten a meal. She noticed new digestive symptoms, such as gas and bloating. From all the travel, she also felt dry and depleted—which are signs of a Vata imbalance. All of this exacerbated the symptoms that she was already experiencing due to menopause.

Dr. Suhas instructed her to make time to come to his clinic for Ayurvedic treatments. Initially, it was a challenge to create the time for a healing immersion, but she knew she had to do something. She received soothing hot-oil massages twice a week, as well as *bastis* (oil enemas) and *nasya* therapy (placing warm oil in the nostrils). From an Ayurvedic perspective, these are therapies that can balance Vata and work in various ways.

Many Ayurvedic treatments work via nervous system regulation, and others provide the physical benefits of hydrating via warm oils, even balancing the digestive tract. In addition to body therapies, Anita added visualization and journaling to her daily routine. She revealed that she had been haunted by thoughts of not being a good daughter, which interfered with her sleep. Before she left, she was given a set of practices to continue after she got home that could fit into her lifestyle. The Vata-balancing routine that she continued at home alleviated her symptoms within a couple of months, and although she suggested that she would take her dad back home to India, she was discouraged from traveling for a while as it could disrupt the breakthroughs she'd made in her health. Because she now understood how the travel affected her overall health, she decided to take her father back at some point in the future.

As her story demonstrates, insomnia often exists in the context of other life circumstances that all need to be addressed. Having our sleep disrupted is like derailing a train—we go off in the wrong direction until we crash. This happens all the time, often due to a gradual accumulation of stress, further compounded when we travel from one continent to another, or even one state to another, which is increasingly common in our modern lives. This disrupts our usual routine, which may be getting us by but eventually catches up to us. When we pay attention to all aspects of our lives, we can avoid derailing the train and stay on track.

PHASES AND SHIFTS: WHY YOUR SLEEP CAN'T CATCH A BREAK

Many of us have unique lifestyle circumstances that affect our sleep during different moments of our lives. Although there are strategies we can adopt in order to meet our sleep challenges exactly where we are, some of us may feel that we have a further distance to walk. In such cases, we encourage you not to do anything too dramatic but to remember that there are many paths to awakened sleep—and taking small steps will still get you to the goal.

Some of our life circumstances are temporary phases while others correspond to longer-term situations that may interfere with our sleep. Let's explore some of these below.

Perimenopause/Menopause

Perimenopause is the transitional period during which menstruation becomes more and more irregular and the body is preparing for menopause, which represents the end of the menstrual cycle. This occurs naturally as the levels of reproductive hormones decline.

Menopause (and in many cases, perimenopause) can be associated with other symptoms as well, such as insomnia, especially in the form of difficulty remaining asleep. Hot flashes and night sweats are known as *vasomotor symptoms* and occur with changes in our blood vessels that influence our body temperature. Vasomotor symptoms afflict people who are menopausal and can be a primary cause of insomnia that can significantly affect quality of life.[8] Managing vasomotor symptoms is key in improving sleep quality, and there are many ways to do this.

Some people may choose to take hormones during this transitional period, which can be effective if there are no medical reasons not to take them. There are other pharmaceuticals besides hormones that can be used as well. However, many of the people we encounter choose not to take hormones or other medications, or they can't due to risk factors. CBT-I can be useful for people who do not wish to take medications. And a recent in-depth review reported that hypnotherapy can be an effective treatment of vasomotor symptoms and can help people sleep by treating this root cause.[9]

Fortunately, there are herbal protocols that have been used for thousands of years that can help with these symptoms. From an Ayurvedic perspective, this transition time, around age fifty, occurs between the

Pitta stage of life (adulthood) to the Vata stage of life (wisdom years), much like the natural transition of summer to fall. Our work with Claudia and Anita, who were both going through menopause, highlights the power of looking to Ayurvedic wisdom to consider the ways we can find soothing sources of balance during the transition between the Pitta and Vata stages of life. As the vasomotor symptoms are primarily a result of Pitta imbalances (which have accumulated over adulthood), a person can look to Pitta-balancing protocols to help with these symptoms. One can also pay attention in their early adult years to reduce Pitta imbalance in their life, so they have less of it in transitional times like menopause.

Being a Night Shift Worker

Night shift (a.k.a. third shift) workers typically begin work in the evening and end in the early morning. Unlike those who work daytime shifts, who are typically aligned with their body's internal clock (the circadian rhythm, which we'll visit in depth in Chapter 3), shift workers are disconnected from the natural cues that let us know it's the right time to sleep. This circadian disruption results in sleep and wakefulness disruption and excessive sleepiness and fatigue.

The Centers for Disease Control's National Health and Nutrition Examination Survey revealed that night shift workers have a significantly higher prevalence of insufficient sleep (less than seven hours) compared to day shift workers.[10] The survey also found that workers who frequently used sleeping pills had a higher prevalence of poor sleep quality, insomnia, and impaired sleep-related activities of daily living, despite adequate sleep time. Excessive sleepiness and poor sleep quality result in an increase in workplace accidents, motor vehicle accidents, and work productivity. Overall, being a night shift worker can bring on drowsiness when it's not wanted, as well as difficulty falling and staying asleep, which can lead to injuries and increase the risk of other health conditions. Unfortunately, night shift workers are also more susceptible to metabolic syndrome, a set of conditions that increase the risk of stroke, heart attack, diabetes, and various forms of cancer, not to mention higher levels of depression and anxiety.[11]

There are ways to manage these risks, including timed light exposure. Other strategies that help are sleeping immediately after a shift by using light-blocking shades, ear plugs, and an eye mask and splitting sleep into two phases of three to four hours. In cases of shift-work sleep issues, a personalized approach is needed to come up with the right plan.

Dr. Suhas recently treated a nurse, Alex, who worked from 7 p.m. to 1 a.m. In order to defuse work-related stress, Alex spent an hour or two watching Netflix before falling asleep. He'd wake up at 10 a.m., eat brunch at noon, scarf down an early dinner at 4 or 5 p.m., and then head to work. He'd drink caffeine all night to stay awake. Knowing that his work schedule wasn't about to change anytime soon, Dr. Suhas suggested that Alex cut out the caffeine and Netflix, do a simple warm-oil self-massage before bed, and change his sleep hours to 1:30–8:30 a.m., which proved to be enough. With some cardio in the morning, he felt more energized than before, and his previous challenges eventually waned.

Being a New Parent

Many new parents, especially mothers, have been through the challenges associated with sleep deprivation. Abrupt shifts in hormone levels, as well as postpartum fatigue and the necessity of attending to an infant around the clock, can have deleterious effects on sleep quantity and quality for months or even years after childbirth. This can have profound impacts on mood and concentration and is linked to postpartum depression— something that is experienced by one in eight women.[12] These postpartum sleep disturbances have been shown to affect fathers as well, with an increased risk of depression for both parents.[13]

Again, an individualized approach is important in these situations, taking into account cultural, social, and personal beliefs. Many people choose to sleep with their child, also known as co-sleeping. This is common among breastfeeding mothers because they can feed at night without getting out of bed or turning on lights. Although controversy abounds on this topic, co-sleeping can be self-regulating for parent(s) and infant, as it supports limbic resonance—the idea that we can experience deep emotional bonding from feelings that are activated by dopamine and norepinephrine, neurotransmitters that regulate stress reactions and the sleep/wake cycle. Co-sleeping has existed in many cultures throughout human history, and it may generate deeper feelings of joy, peace, and security. That said, there is data and concern regarding an increased risk of sudden infant death syndrome (SIDS), so the American Academy of Pediatrics recommends room sharing instead, where the infant sleeps in the same room as the parent but not in the same bed.

Regardless of sleep arrangements, sleep disruption during this time period occurs for all groups, and management needs to be done on a case-by-case basis. During her decade of providing prenatal, obstetric, and postpartum care to patients of many different belief systems and socioeconomic levels, Dr. Sheila recognized the importance of working with each family to find the right solution. Many families have strong opinions about the right approach for their infants, and although science can guide us, it can't give us the right answer for each person.

Although studies on the postpartum period are lacking, some strategies that help other populations can help sleepy parents as well. These include meditation, yoga, tai chi, and other practices that induce the relaxation response. A common recommendation is to "sleep when the baby sleeps." A study published in 2023 in the journal *Sleep* showed support for daytime napping and a correlation between regular daytime sleep and the prevention of postpartum depression.[14]

Frequent Travel and Changes in Time Zone

Both of us have worked with patients who travel regularly for work as well as for pleasure. Unsurprisingly, frequently moving across time zones is extremely disruptive. The body clock regulates our functions while we're both sleeping and waking. Plane travel may be convenient, but it puts us out of sync with our body clock. Although jet lag is temporary when our travel schedule is infrequent, it can be disruptive to our circadian rhythm when travel is baked into our lifestyle.

Although frequent travel is one of the consequences of living in a globalized world, both of us have a lot of experience helping patients to mitigate its impacts. Our common tips to our globetrotting patients include several Ayurvedic practices to balance the Vata aggravation (excessive change, movement, and dryness) that occurs with travel. These can be started a few days prior to travel and include oil massage and nasya, nasal oil drops, which calm the Vata dosha and help keep body rhythms regular. It's also a good idea to eat warm, moist foods during travel. We recommend avoiding the commonly served cold drinks while traveling (you can ask for hot water on an airplane and take calming herbal tea bags with you). In addition, spending time outside in your new environment can reset your ability to fall asleep, so getting sunlight during the day in the place where you land helps regulate your internal clock more quickly.

In general, keeping a regular schedule while in your travel location will also help your sleep schedule. We advise against chugging caffeine to stay awake for an early meeting after a red-eye flight, because this will disrupt your sleep as well as your ability to easily adjust to your new time zone. Although that jolt of caffeine can create alertness and even improve your cognition temporarily,[15] it can also lead to a caffeine crash. Caffeine acts in part by blocking receptors for the neurotransmitter adenosine.[16] Adenosine naturally builds up over the day and binds to receptors in the brain. After about twelve to sixteen hours, as it peaks, it suppresses wakefulness and promotes drowsiness. However, as caffeine is eliminated from your system, the adenosine that has been produced binds the receptors all at once and creates the "crash" that occurs after caffeine intake. This sleepiness can interfere with the activities you have planned for your work or leisure schedule.

Many of us will find ways to accommodate life phases and circumstances like the ones we've just noted, but we can do so only up to a certain point. Overall, as we learn to train ourselves to sync up with our circadian rhythm, even small changes can take us far.

DOSHA DRAMA: WHAT'S THROWING YOUR BALANCE OFF?

One of the causes of disrupted sleep patterns is an accumulation of any one of the doshas. Typically, one or more factors in your life will cause the qualities of a specific dosha to accumulate, to the point that it's aggravated and causes symptoms. From an Ayurvedic perspective, like increases like. So, more dryness, cold, lightness, irregularity, and movement will cause a Vata imbalance. Too much heat, focus, intensity, and overdoing will create a Pitta imbalance. Immobility, as well as cold, wet, heavy qualities will lead to a Kapha imbalance. These dosha qualities can accumulate due to experiences or choices in any area of life, be it food, exercise, work, or relationships.

Remember that everyone has all three doshas as they are all needed to carry out the functions in the body, so any one of them can get out of balance. Whenever there is an aggravation of any of the doshas, we will be affected in some way. All this comes into play with sleep, as in all aspects of life. So, even though your constitution might be that of a Pitta, or a medium sleeper, you could actually be in a state of Vata imbalance due to frequent travel, which may look like going through a spell of light sleeping and frequent awakening due to the Vata accumulation in your body. Or that same Pitta person who normally wakes up with a bright mind could develop heaviness and moisture if they've been eating cold foods or eating too late at night—or even if the weather has been cold and wet. This can then cause nasal congestion and feelings of sluggishness in the morning—signs of a Kapha imbalance. Paying attention to which qualities are out of balance gives you a clue as to which dosha needs balancing.

Depending on our innate body type, the same dosha imbalance can look different for each individual, so it's important to connect to what is happening in *you*, not someone else. We once worked with a couple, Mike and Helen. Helen was a Vata and Mike was a Kapha. They went on a cruise to Alaska in the summer, where they were subject to the rocking of the boat as well as longer daylight hours. The accumulation of light and movement made it more challenging than usual for Helen to fall asleep. Within seven days, she'd lost three pounds because she had no appetite and wasn't sleeping well. In contrast, Mike didn't mind the sensation of being rocked to sleep (his superpower is sleep, after all) and felt energized by the long days. This goes to show that you might have the same experience, but depending on your dosha, you'll respond differently!

Because the doshas express themselves differently in each person, it's a good idea to look more deeply at how certain dosha aggravations may be playing out in our own lives. Typically, if we're experiencing a Vata imbalance, this can show up as cold hands and feet, a tendency toward restless legs or muscle spasms, pain in the body, bloating, gas, dehydration, overactive mind and nervous system, palpitations, anxiety, and a general sense of spaciness. A Pitta imbalance may look like heartburn, indigestion, thirst in the middle of the night, difficulty quieting the mind (especially in a time of intense work), overthinking or overplanning, irritability, a tendency to overheat, or skin issues. A Kapha imbalance might show up as weight gain or difficulty losing weight, a feeling of constant fullness, excessive sleepiness, low metabolism and digestion, sluggishness, fluid retention, feeling depressed or stuck, and a general lack of motivation.

Please remember that these are all generalized statements as dosha aggravations vary depending on your unique body type. Many times, there are multiple imbalances occurring at once (just as a storm can be windy, hot, and rainy all at the same time!). The important thing to note is that dosha aggravations can be very disruptive to your sleep—but based on the symptoms you're experiencing, it's possible to turn to a balancing regimen that will help mitigate and reduce the excessive presence of any particular dosha.

ASSESSMENT: WHICH DOSHA IS KEEPING YOU UP AT NIGHT?

The assessment at the end of Chapter 1 helped you understand your primary dosha in the context of your overall lifetime sleep tendencies. For example, if you had more Vata/light sleeper responses than Pitta/medium sleeper or Kapha/deep sleeper responses, you will primarily be looking for a balancing regimen that characterizes Vata, your dominant dosha.

However, it's possible to experience an imbalance that corresponds to the doshas that are *not* predominant for you. In such a case, you might have excess Pitta or Kapha. It's possible to have multiple imbalances, but the assessment below will help you be more conscious of the imbalance that could be affecting your current sleep difficulties right now. Recall from Chapter 1, this is known as vikruti, or your current imbalance. As the seasons and circumstances of your life change, so will your dosha imbalances, so be sure to answer the questions based on what you're experiencing in your life today.

This assessment will help you identify the dosha imbalances that could be affecting you at this time. Just like the questions at the end of Chapter 1, all answers will be in a yes/no format. Give yourself a score of 1 for all "yes" answers, and 0 for all "no" answers.

Sleep Sensitivity (Vata Imbalance)

1. Do you have difficulty falling asleep due to worries and anxiety?
2. Do you wake up during the night due to restlessness or feeling too cold?
3. Do you respond to a poor night's sleep by feeling tired and restless the next day?
4. Does a poor night's sleep make you anxious and affect your mood?

Score: _____

Restless Sleep (Pitta Imbalance)

1. Do you fall asleep but wake up in the middle of the night thinking about your to-do list?
2. Do you wake up feeling hot in the middle of the night?
3. Does a poor night's sleep make you irritable and grumpy the next day?
4. Does a poor night's sleep affect your ability to focus and concentrate the next day?

Score: _____

Heavy Sleep (Kapha Imbalance)

1. Do you fall asleep easily but have difficulty waking up?
2. Do you snore during the night or wake up with congestion?
3. Does a poor night's sleep make you drowsy and tired the next day?

4. Does a poor night's sleep influence your mood by making you feel heavy and depressed?

Score: _____

Once you've determined your score, you'll have a sense of where you may have a current dosha imbalance. Again, it's possible to have more than one imbalance. In addition, the imbalance you are having now may be different from your natural sleep tendencies. You can start by balancing the one that is most out of balance, or try practices that can balance two doshas at the same time (for example, warmth can balance both Vata and Kapha, slowing down can balance both Vata and Pitta, and reducing oils in the diet can balance both Pitta and Kapha). Pay attention to which qualities you've accumulated as this will help you incorporate stabilizing routines for both your prakruti (natural constitution) and vikruti (current imbalances).

REFLECTIONS

1. With respect to the three pillars of well-being, how is your sleep currently being affected (e.g., by physiological issues, mental/emotional factors, overall quality of life and connection to spiritual meaning, or a combination of all three)?
2. Have you used or are you presently using any sleep aids (such as melatonin, prescription medication, alcohol, etc.) to self-medicate? How have these affected you?
3. How would you describe your sleep? Is it high-quality, low-quality, or somewhere in between?
4. If you've had sleep challenges, how long have they been going on? Often, although we tend to think of them as "just the way it is," our sleep habits are usually carried over from a young age—in

other words, they aren't natural to our constitution but, rather, learned and replicated over the years.

5. Are sleep challenges something you've come to accept, or something you're willing to shift with the practices and recommendations in this book? Please remember that, as you incorporate our practices into your sleep regimen, you may find that you aren't quite as dependent on the things that used to help you sleep! We also encourage you to set an intention to bring awareness to your thoughts and activities throughout the day as this can shed light on your sleep issues and steer you in the direction of healthier choices.

List any takeaways from this chapter that you'd like to incorporate into your own sleep-hygiene routine:

_____

_____

_____

_____

_____

CHAPTER 3

) ◗ ● ◖ (

WHAT HAPPENS
WHEN WE SLEEP?

Finish each day before you begin the next, and
interpose a solid wall of sleep between the two.

—Ralph Waldo Emerson

WE HAVE A BASIC UNDERSTANDING THAT SLEEP IS ESSENTIAL. AT the same time, it remains cloaked in mystery—in other words, we don't really know *why* we do it, even though all animals need some form of rest or sleep. But scientific study hasn't yet determined *why* sleep takes up a third of our life, and *why* it wreaks such havoc on our well-being when we don't manage to get it.

Obviously, sleep affects the many facets of our overall health. Some scientists think it's an evolutionary process to conserve energy, restore and clear metabolites (small molecules that are intermediate products of our metabolism—including amino acids, lipids, and sugars), and promote brain health. However, the true purpose of sleep can't be totally understood without addressing its psychospiritual nature—which is hard to explain in a purely materialist framework but is the basis of how we experience the most important aspects of our lives.

However, traditional Eastern perspectives give us a deeper explanation of sleep and why it's so integral to our overall health. The *Charaka Samhita*, an ancient Ayurvedic text, notes that too little, too much, or erratic sleep can all negatively affect our essential life force, leading to a weakened mind and body. Ayurveda and Vedic wisdom point to sleep as a powerful curative that can rejuvenate us on every level. Sleep is one of the most pivotal experiences we can have, as it allows us to more easily access consciousness, which is the source of healing. As our external sensory experience fades, we have the capacity to come face-to-face with our infinite, creative nature, which is outside of space and time and the rules of the material world (which is why we can fly in our dreams!). Vedic wisdom isn't alone here. Plenty of other ancient systems, including traditional Chinese medicine, have noted that there's a lot more than physical healing and restoration that's taking place as we sleep.

Although Western science has defined particular states of sleep, such as light sleep, deep sleep, and dream sleep, it is unclear as to the benefits of other sleep states that we experience. One such example is hypnagogic sleep, the transitional state between waking and sleep. In this state, alpha waves, which mark our waking state, decrease considerably, but we're still not asleep. The same is true for the hypnopompic state, when we transition from sleep to waking. Similarly, the purpose of dreaming (which takes place during REM sleep) is shrouded in mystery, although there are plenty of theories. Once again, Vedic wisdom offers answers that live beyond the materialist framework, pointing to the possibility of mystical states that may visit us only when we dream.

In this chapter, we'll offer some insight into what Western science *does* know about sleep from an objective and scientific perspective (as well as what researchers are still attempting to put together), and combine that with some food for thought as to what the ancients knew and understood regarding why good sleep is integral to what might be its higher purpose: maintaining a state of balance with the natural rhythms of life and allowing us to access our limitless selves. Our hope is that you'll walk away with a more complete, nuanced vision of the "why" behind sleep, as well as how sleep connects us to larger cycles to which we intrinsically belong.

HOW AND WHEN WE DRIFT OFF

Nighttime sleep is primarily induced by the interplay of two hormones, melatonin and cortisol. The main stimulus for the rise in melatonin in the evening is darkness. A small area of the brain called the suprachiasmatic nucleus senses darkness and signals the pineal gland to release melatonin into the system. Rising melatonin suppresses cortisol (the hormone of wakefulness and alertness), binds to melatonin receptors in the brain, and makes us feel drowsy. It increases over several hours and peaks in the middle of the night, before it slowly starts to decrease so we can awaken. Meanwhile, cortisol starts to rise in the later part of the night, around 2–3 a.m., and peaks around 8:30 a.m.

With exposure to sunlight upon waking, melatonin production drops significantly and there is a significant rise in the level of cortisol, which makes us feel awake. In the past, human sleep patterns were more in sync with the rising and setting sun; however, in our modern environment, we interrupt natural sleep cycles with artificial light, especially blue light from our screens. It's important for our physiology to maintain normal levels of melatonin at night as it's not only a hormone that enables sleep but has also been found to regulate blood pressure, reproductive functions, and metabolism.

Nonrestorative sleep at night can create drowsiness during the day. And since our normal physiology creates a period of decreased alertness in the afternoon, we can feel especially drowsy if we aren't sleeping at night. While some studies show that a nap can be restorative, others suggest it can interfere with falling asleep at night. Still other studies suggest that longer daytime naps may end up increasing inflammatory markers and cortisol levels to the extent that this could lead to insulin resistance, as well as the accumulation of visceral fat.[1] And although there is some data that catch-up sleep can help to reduce some of this inflammation, the data is not definitive. The jury's still out, scientifically speaking, on whether naps are good for us or not. But of course, there is no one-size-fits-all answer, even when it comes to naps. In fact, research is showing us there may be a genetic component to daytime napping. A study done using the UK Biobank identified dozens of gene regions associated with napping. The researchers suggest that future work in this area may help to better personalize napping recommendations.[2]

According to Ayurveda, there can be benefits to napping, but that depends on the context. Ayurveda has always suggested a personalized approach to sleep recommendations. For example, Vata (light sleeper) types are usually advised to nap after lunch for about thirty minutes if possible, even though it may be hard for them to slow down. This is especially true if they're older, as Vata types (especially in the Vata stage of life) can expend energy quickly and feel exhausted. In contrast, Kaphas (deep sleepers) are instructed not to nap, since movement and activity are what keeps them in balance—although a Kapha would love to take a nap anytime. Again, we look to the wisdom of using opposite qualities to achieve balance, even with napping.

Illness can also naturally induce sleep, of course. Production of white blood cells, which fight infection, increases when we're sick. This acute inflammatory response releases proteins, including cytokines and prostaglandins, both of which support the immune system in fighting off infection and play a role in the regulation of sleep. Although the mechanisms are quite complex, it's clear that this immune–brain crosstalk allows us to rest and conserve energy during illness. In addition to immune proteins, bacterial and viral cell components that are released as germs are destroyed can also trigger sleepiness. Most of us recognize we're more tired during illness—and when we rest, it's easier to heal from an acute infection.

In science, we describe the molecules that induce sleep and some of the factors that can affect their production or activity. However, Ayurveda describes sleep induction in a different way. The *Charaka Samhita* talks about seven primary types of sleep. One key type arises from the healthy exhaustion of the senses after a day of balanced activity. In this state, the sense organs naturally disentangle from their objects of perception after a day of healthy activity, allowing the mind to withdraw inward. This process of sensory unwinding characterizes good sleep, enabling deep restoration and rejuvenation. When our sense organs unwind from external stimuli, we get to go within and enjoy restorative sleep.

The process of the sense organs naturally withdrawing from their objects of perception, allowing the body and mind to rest and rejuvenate, is known as *pratyahara*. Why is this so integral to good sleep? Because throughout the day, our sense organs—eyes, ears, nose, tongue, and skin—are constantly engaged with external stimuli, creating subtle attachments to the objects of our sensory perception. As we prepare for sleep, disengagement is necessary so we can turn inward and the nervous system can recalibrate. This process allows the body to repair itself and integrate daily experiences. Overstimulation can interfere with the practice of pratyahara, which is why calming evening rituals are so crucial for promoting deep, restful sleep.

The text also notes that good sleep in quality and quantity leads to happiness, nourishment, strength, knowledge, and life itself. On the other side, excessive, irregular, or poor sleep can lead to unhappiness, depletion, weakness, disease, and a reduced lifespan. Proper sleep helps us to ensure that our doshas remain in equilibrium, which enables us to maintain all aspects of our health. In contrast, inadequate sleep can increase Vata, which leads to a wasting away of our tissues, as well as degenerative conditions and restlessness of the mind. On the other end, oversleep leads to an increase in Kapha and can result in obesity and chronic diseases such as diabetes.

According to Ayurveda, the types of sleep are influenced by what's happening in the mind and body. Each type has a root cause, some of which have correlates in modern science as well:

1. **Mind-dulling slumber** is a sleep that's influenced by *tamas*, which is one of three energetic qualities known as the *gunas*, according to Vedic wisdom. Tamas represents darkness, illusion, and ignorance. This type of sleep is characterized by mind-dulling forms of passive entertainment—such as alcohol, mind-altering substances, heavy and impure foods, or watching TV or videos on our phone in order to lull ourselves into a stupor. Generally, when we attempt to induce this kind of sleep, there's an artificial quality to it, such that we end up feeling dull but not rested.

2. **Food-induced slumber** occurs when we eat Kapha-aggravating foods, including dairy or heavy carbs, or when we eat too late at night. We might have no problem getting to sleep, but we'll usually have difficulty waking up because of the accumulation of *ama*, a Sanskrit word that describes unmetabolized waste in the body, usually from undigested foods—which can end up causing a Kapha aggravation that compromises our quality of sleep over time.

3. **Exertion-induced slumber** occurs when we push ourselves to our mental and physical limits—we work too hard, we play too hard, we have a hectic schedule, and we take in too much stimulation. Our senses are fatigued, which can lead to feeling both tired and wired. Ideally, we should feel pleasantly exhausted when falling asleep, but overexertion can make us achy, restless, and unable to cultivate the relaxation that's necessary to drift off.

4. **Externally induced slumber** is caused by external factors outside our control—such as accidents, bereavement, the use of

medicines, odors in our environment, or any physical or mental trauma that leads to an acute reaction that triggers the onset of sleep. Essentially, an external influence has affected our mind, body, or both.

5. **Illness-induced slumber** occurs when our body fights off disease and illness, including colds and infections. This is actually a positive form of sleep because it's healing and boosts our immunity. Sleeping for several hours during the day when we're sick can enable us to recover from chronic diseases and imbalances.

6. **Natural slumber** is the nighttime sleep that's associated with our natural circadian rhythm. It's in sync with nature's light and darkness cycles.

7. **Death slumber** is the state of our fading consciousness as we prepare for the ultimate journey from this world into the next. This type of sleep occurs only when we're close to death—hinging between consciousness and what's on the other side. Interestingly, the Sanskrit term is *kaala swabhava prasava*, which translates to "natural childbirth"! It's as if the ancient sages saw this period as a liminal time during which we reenter the nurturing womb of consciousness in preparation for the next phase of our adventure.

Ayurveda is clear about the importance of sleep. Life and death are thought to be entirely dependent on the quality of our sleep, which is why it's a system that focuses on ways we can demonstrably improve our sleep rather than striving to objectively measure the mechanisms and details that fuel it.

Whatever paradigm we look at—Western science or Vedic wisdom—it is clear that the reasons we sleep and the mechanisms behind sleep are varied. They range from normal, healthy, restorative sleep all the way to dysregulated, nonrestorative sleep. When we live a healthy, balanced lifestyle and prevent disease, we can develop more of the type of sleep that is healing and restorative.

NREM AND REM SLEEP: THE DYNAMIC DUO OF SLEEP

In Western science, sleep is described as a state of reduced responsiveness, motor activity, and metabolism that's divided into two phases: rapid eye movement (REM) and non–rapid eye movement (NREM). Each phase has various stages. The body cycles through these two phases four to six times a night, with each combined cycle of NREM and REM lasting an average of 90–120 minutes. We spend 75–80 percent of our time in the stages of NREM sleep. A REM sleep cycle always follows NREM sleep, and most REM sleep occurs in the second half of the night. Several factors can influence the time we spend in each phase, though, such as aging, physical and mental health conditions, medications, and sleep-stage disorders.

NREM takes us from wakefulness to deep sleep. As we fall asleep, our brain activity, breathing, and heart rate slow as our body temperature dips and our muscles relax. NREM sleep is deeply restorative, as it's a time during which our tissues are rebuilt and repaired, bone and muscle are built, and our immune system gets to hit the reset button.

In REM sleep, the eyes rapidly move in different directions without sending visual details to the brain. Dreams most often occur during REM, although they're also possible in NREM.

Let's briefly look at the stages of NREM and REM sleep.

NREM

- **Stage N1:** Falling asleep—heartbeat and breathing slow down and muscles relax, which lasts a few minutes. This stage normally accounts for about 5 percent of total sleep time.

- **Stage N2:** Light sleep—heartbeat and breathing continue to slow, eye movement wanes, and body temperature is reduced. This stage lasts about twenty-five minutes and lengthens with each cycle over the night, making up about 45 percent of sleep time.
- **Stage N3:** Slow-wave/deep sleep—heartbeat and breathing are extremely slow, eye movement stops, and the body is fully relaxed. Our response to external stimuli is reduced. In this stage, we experience cell regeneration, detoxification, tissue repair, and the strengthening of our immune system. The glymphatic system of the brain is most active during this phase, clearing out waste and toxins.[3] This stage lasts about twenty to forty minutes and accounts for 25 percent of total sleep time. This is such a deep sleep state that if someone is abruptly awakened from it, they're likely to feel foggy and groggy for some time afterward. Sleepwalking, night terrors, and bedwetting can occur at this stage. As we age, we have less time in this stage, and more time in stage N2—unfortunately, lack of N3 has been shown to increase the risk of dementia.[4]

REM

REM sleep makes up 25 percent of our time asleep, but the first stage we experience during the night is only about ten minutes. As we progress through the night, each REM cycle increases until it reaches about an hour. People typically awaken in the morning during REM sleep and may remember the dream they were just having.

REM is the primary dreaming stage of sleep—and the time when our eye movements become rapid, our breath and heart rate increase, our brain activity increases, and our limbs are temporarily paralyzed. Presumably, the paralysis kicks in so we don't act out the content of our dreams. The brain is so active at this time that our brain metabolism increases by about 20 percent![5]

Although it used to be believed that we don't dream during NREM, this isn't true. However, many researchers suggest that our dreams are a lot less vivid and sensorily rich in NREM than in REM . . . which may be another good reason for limb paralysis during REM!

However, after so many decades, there are still many questions left unanswered in modern sleep science as to the true essence and purpose of REM sleep. Many sleep researchers are currently questioning the way REM sleep is classified, and they agree that this stage of sleep is filled with perplexities and paradoxes we can't fully explain.[6] We know that without REM sleep, our capacity to learn, consolidate knowledge, and develop memory would all be hindered. Overall, life with a reduced REM sleep duration isn't ideal.[7] In fact, a study in *JAMA Neurology* in 2020 showed a lack of proper REM sleep in adults was associated with an increased risk of all-cause mortality, or death.[8]

Another thing to note here is that while so much of the information we have about the sleep stages comes from electroencephalogram (EEG) measurements of brain waves, these measurements take into account activity only in the cerebral cortex of the brain, not in deeper brain structures. However, research is revealing that different parts of the brain may be going through different sleep stages at the same time. Essentially, even if the cerebral cortex is awake, other parts of our brain might be asleep.

Dr. Sheila once had an eighteen-year-old patient who came to her with signs of chronic insomnia. "I don't sleep—in fact, I'm awake all night," he told her. "If I sleep, it might be for an hour, and then I wake up." However, the disruption in his sleep didn't show up in his grades. In fact, he was a straight A student! Although he did struggle with fatigue and poor moods, it seemed that parts of his brain had adapted in such a way that his focus and concentration weren't affected at all.

Could it be that, even when his cerebral cortex was subjected to long hours of awakeness, other parts of his brain were compensating by falling asleep and receiving the benefits of restoration and learning? And could this be a capacity that we can consciously control? There are several references in Vedic mythology of adepts (highly skilled yogis) who did not require sleep or required very little sleep. Perhaps the yogis understood something more about controlling different parts of the brain, even during wakefulness, than modern science does.

Overall, stories like these demonstrate that more research is needed to understand sleep from a scientific perspective. Then again, there may be aspects of sleep that defy measurement. Thankfully, the Vedic perspective can supplement our understanding in powerful ways.

GROOVE TO YOUR CIRCADIAN BEAT

The term *circadian* comes from the Latin *circa* ("around") and *dia* ("day")—literally translating to "around the day," which is why most people refer to the circadian rhythm as our daily body clock. This is the rhythmic activity that occurs within every cell of the body over the course of a day. It's a twenty-four-hour cycle that comprises the internal clock of the body and holds court over our most essential functions and processes, including hormone release, digestion, and body temperature—all of which influence our sleep and wakefulness. The circadian rhythm is primarily regulated by the suprachiasmatic nucleus, which is affected by light and darkness; however, the circadian rhythm within individual cells is also affected by food intake and physical activity, among other things.

Sleep research naturally involves circadian-rhythm research as circadian rhythms give us a clear picture of our physical and psychological cycles throughout the twenty-four hours of day and night and are a primary regulator of sleep cycles. While most agree that sleep *quantity* is important for the majority of us, a recent study notes that sleep *regularity*, with consistent timing around our sleeping and waking, is a much stronger predictor of mortality risk than the number of hours of sleep.[9] When we artificially disrupt this regularity by even an hour, as in modern society's adoption of daylight saving time, our body notices. This can result in circadian misalignment and worsened mood, as well as an increase in cardiovascular events and car crashes, to the extent that the American Academy of Sleep Medicine has recommended abandoning this practice.[10] Ayurveda also supports the idea that going to bed and waking up at the same time every day serves us well in the long term, especially since a regular schedule helps to keep the irregular nature of Vata in balance. In fact, the entire concept of the circadian rhythm maps onto the concept of the daily Ayurvedic dosha clock, which we'll explore in detail later in the chapter.

Ayurveda takes the concept of natural rhythms a step further than just a day, noting that aside from the twenty-four-hour rhythm, we also have a seasonal rhythm that occurs over the twelve months of our year. In fact, Ayurveda ascribes many diseases to the seasonal aggravation of specific doshas—which is why, with every seasonal change, Ayurvedic doctors will prescribe protocols that address the accumulation of certain doshas, including seasonal detoxification and rejuvenation.

From an Ayurvedic perspective, we have natural spontaneous urges known as *vegas*—which include the urge to sleep or eat and occur at specific times of the day. When they are suppressed or get out of sync, we can become very sick. For example, something as seemingly harmless as jet lag can interfere with our digestive urges, causing us to have bowel movements at erratic times or suppressing our appetite. Every time you relinquish an urge, especially as natural as the one to sleep, it becomes more difficult to welcome it back. This is why many people who suppress the urge to sleep when it comes on have difficulty falling asleep later. If we don't pay attention to our vegas, our entire physiology can be thrown off. From an Ayurvedic perspective, a vega is like a rising wave, and we need to catch the wave at the top in order to get to where we need to go. When we don't, we create an imbalance in the body.

In addition to the health risks that Ayurveda associates with suppressed vegas, an irregular lifestyle can also lead to the excess of a particular dosha in the body. We can create an imbalance in any three of the doshas for a variety of reasons, but when we suppress a vega, we are suppressing the movement of energy in the body, causing Vata dosha to accumulate. This can ultimately lead to symptoms of a Vata imbalance, such as disrupted, irregular sleep.

Our sleep cycles can also be disrupted when we experience a dosha aggravation caused by seasonal transitions. As the Earth rotates around the sun, we experience specific shifts in qualities that dominate outside in nature, and within us. Our physiology is affected, just as it is for plants and animals. Using a typical four-season climate as an example, the Vata dosha will accumulate and get out of balance in the cool, dry months of early autumn through early winter, which can affect sleep. Pitta can accumulate during the late spring through late summer, when there's a danger of overheating. Kapha can accumulate in the later months of winter, as well as the early spring—when there is melting snow and rain, leading to congestion. The accumulation of these qualities can all lead to disrupted sleep if we are not adjusting our lifestyle practices to accommodate the changing qualities of nature. And when we don't address or balance these seasonal dosha accumulations, they can often lead to diseases. Just as nature goes through cycles, so does our physiology—which means we need to be aware of what doshas are accumulating throughout the seasons and develop practices to keep them balanced.

The diagram below shows the dominant dosha in each of the typical four-season climate regions of the world. Keep in mind that the dominant dosha can vary depending on the seasons in different parts of the world. To know which dosha is accumulating, simply consider the qualities of the air outside; feel the temperature and humidity, and

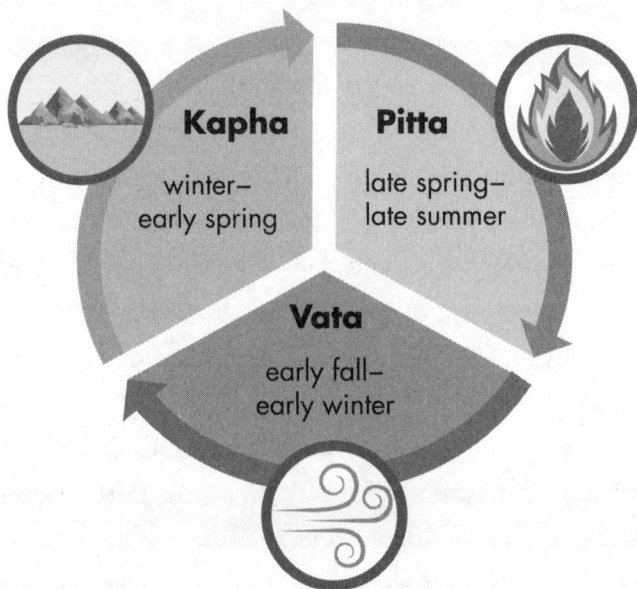

you will know which doshas predominate and can increase in your body.

Beyond the seasons, Ayurveda also points to the monthly lunar rhythms of the moon, which exert an influence over the tides, as well as our menstrual cycles and cholesterol metabolism.[11] The monthly lunar cycle may even influence drowsiness, sleep habits, moods, and the secretion of hormones that are integral to our sleep/wake cycle.[12]

In addition, Ayurveda recognizes the subtle effects of the celestial rhythms of the planets. The *Srimad Bhagavatam* is a Vedic text that describes cosmic cycles and colossal passages of time—which determines what's known as the *kalachakra*, or the cosmic wheel of time on which everything in existence pivots. The Ayurvedic concept of the body clock describes the way our cells are capable of tracking the movement of the sun, moon, stars, and galaxies to create our perception of time.

We have rhythms within rhythms within rhythms, some obvious and some more subtle. So, it's no surprise that the more we seek answers about our biological cycles, the more complexity we discover. Yet, when we become more intimately connected to the seasons and cycles of our lives, we can tell the time of day without glancing at a clock—even if we're indoors. Often, this is the case with our patients who come to learn the methods of awakened sleep.

When it comes to natural rhythms, including circadian rhythms, it's as if our bodies are time machines, and these micro and macro cycles of time are actually embedded in our genes. In fact, research has identified the existence of clock genes, which express the internal timekeeping mechanism that guides our physiology along the rhythms of time.[13] Essentially, at the level of our genes, our bodies are designed to be well attuned to everything that's happening outside our window. What this means, according to Ayurveda, is that when we attempt to go against the grain of these cycles, we interrupt our deeply rooted inclination to follow suit with the rest of nature. The discovery of clock genes highlights and validates the importance of the ancient Ayurvedic principle of a daytime routine (*dinacharya*), nighttime routine (*ratricharya*), and seasonal-change routine (*ritucharya*).

The human body has braved all kinds of environmental adaptations, mostly owing to our own technology and cultural habits, but we are still susceptible to circadian disruptions that can affect our health, and in highly individualized ways. For example, Vata types are the most sensitive to sleep disruptions (and disruptions in general) and usually get the best quality of sleep if they go to bed by 10 p.m.; they typically need somewhere between eight and nine hours of sleep to feel their best, while others' doshas may be more resilient to sleep deprivation. In fact, in one study, researchers found that there are distinct variations in several genes between individuals that have "high vulnerability" versus "high resistance" to sleep deprivation.[14] From an Ayurvedic perspective, knowing someone's dosha predicts vulnerability to irregular sleep patterns and sleep deprivation. Predictably, Vata types are more vulnerable, and Pitta and Kapha types are more resilient to sleep deprivation. No doubt we will someday be able to validate these Ayurvedic observations with an increased understanding of specific gene patterns related to doshas.

Whatever your primary dosha, daily self-renewal is enhanced by strong physical and emotional digestive systems—and we strengthen these systems by harmonizing our lifestyles with our natural rhythms, which move in recurring cycles of rest and activity with nature. Despite the twists and turns in life that might make us resistant to the idea of keeping in lockstep with nature, chronobiology is, more or less, hardwired into us. When we harmonize with nature, and thus with our true selves, we experience more restorative sleep and better health in general. It's this awakened sleep that helps us make the most of our waking hours.

MORNING PERSON, NIGHT PERSON

Our patients often say, "I know it's probably a good idea for me to fall asleep early and wake up early, but I can't! My spouse is a morning person, but I'm a night person. Is this something I really have any control over?"

The concept of being more or less awake at certain times of the day, and of benefiting from a specific bedtime, is known as a *chronotype*. In shorthand, we tend to reduce chronotypes to either an early bird or a night owl. Most of us are a mixture of the two.[15] There are also sleep specialists who have identified not just one but four chronotypes: those who struggle more with sleep in general; those who wake up alert and ready to tackle the day; those who naturally sleep long hours and feel a bit groggy in the morning; and those who feel more alive at night. According to many sleep specialists, chronotypes aren't just about when you go to sleep and when you wake up; they're more about when you tend to function best. For example, early birds feel at their sharpest early in the day, whereas night owls have more energy toward the end of the day.

As there seems to be some genetic regulation of sleep types, it's different strokes for different folks, you could say—but it's also not that simple. Some studies think the idea of being an early bird or a night owl is more of a conditioned response that may not always work to our benefit. The tendency in both Ayurveda and sleep research is to err on the side of "early to bed, early to rise," which supports our circadian rhythm.

A chronotype describes a behavioral pattern we've developed over time more than it does a natural, ingrained one. In other words, it's not rigid or deterministic. It may have evolved from our lifestyle. For example, if we work in an industry that requires us to have meetings and social engagements into the wee hours, it's likely that we'll feel like more of a night owl. Our inner clock adjusts to help us adapt to the situation, and sometimes it does so pretty well.

For example, it was once fairly common throughout the world for humans to sleep biphasically, or with two major sleep periods in a night. The "first sleep" usually took place shortly after sunset, for four hours or so, from about 7 to 11 p.m. That's because it was more difficult to work in the absence of sunlight, so it was more prudent to sleep. Then, from 11 p.m. to midnight or 1 a.m., people would wake up to do light chores around the house or socialize with friends and family around the fire. They would then have their "second sleep" from midnight to 4 a.m., or 1–5 a.m., still waking up before the rooster crowed. All this was the norm prior to the advent of the light bulb, which allowed people to work later and afforded them greater freedom to split their time however they wanted to.[16]

In other cultures, the climate dictated sleep patterns. In many regions of the world, cultural norms around midday naps developed due to the climate. It's not unusual for people in warm climates to take a nap in the middle of the day when it's too hot to work, and resume activity into the evening hours.

Particularly in our modern life, we tend to pattern our lives after learned tendencies that align with shifts in technology or social norms. Modern technology has resulted in adaptable internal clocks. However, when given the opportunity, we will naturally sync to nature's seasonal circadian rhythms. A pivotal 2017 study, known as the "camp study," discovered that even night owls went to bed earlier and slept longer when immersed in nature.[17] The researchers took test subjects out into the Colorado wilderness to camp, and everyone was subjected to the same cycle of light and darkness. The study subsequently showed that our rhythms can shift in as quickly as one weekend. We're ultimately wired to sync to nature's daily and seasonal rhythms.

It does seem to be the case that our body goes through a natural cycle, such that when we get enough exposure to daylight, our nighttime sleep is better—and we actually *want* to go to sleep during the night. But location makes all the difference. There are populations that need to make adjustments when the shift between day and night is dramatic. When Dr. Sheila lived in Southeast Alaska, which experiences close to twenty-four hours of daylight during the summer months, some of her patients found it hard to sleep when it was still light out, so it was also hard to wake up and follow a typical nine-to-five workday. To accommodate for this, many people used heavy light-blocking curtains so they could sleep at the appropriate time. And during the winter months, when twenty-four-hour darkness prevails, it was challenging to wake up and feel energized. The lack of light left many people feeling down or depressed (a phenomenon known as seasonal affective disorder, or SAD). In this situation, they could spend time under UV light or with light-therapy boxes to feel better and avoid depression during the winter months. And other people who did not need to conform to the social clocks of a 9–5 workday utilized the sun during the summer to work on their gardens (which produced a lot in the summer!) and rested more during the winter months.

Speaking of location, we have to keep in mind the social clock of different cultures, which can have just as big an influence over our daily flow as our circadian rhythms do. For example, in cultures across Southern Europe and the Mediterranean, as well as Latin America, families might eat dinner later in the night. So, what happens when your social time doesn't match up with your circadian time? Again, there is no right or wrong here as so many of our behaviors are dictated by adaptations we make, depending on lifestyle and culture. However, our clinical experience has demonstrated, across the board, that it's a good idea to align our internal circadian clock with our social clock for the maximum benefits to our health . . . and the smoothest segue into awakened sleep.

THE DOSHA CLOCK: AYURVEDA'S GUIDE TO YOUR PERFECT SLEEP SCHEDULE

Ayurveda teaches us how to pay attention to nature's cycles so we can create a lifestyle that optimizes our sleep and overall health. It essentially guides us to do the right thing at the right time in accordance with the changes we experience in nature. Ayurveda poetically states that the body is like a blooming lotus that opens during the daylight hours and shuts at nighttime.

Traditionally, Ayurveda has always pointed to the *dosha clock* as a way to ensure that our activities throughout the day are in alignment with natural cycles, as physiological processes are most optimal at certain times of the day. Which processes are occurring at what times, and the ideal times for our daily and nightly activities, can be explained through an understanding of the dosha clock. This clock is broken up into six four-hour zones throughout a twenty-four-hour period, and each dosha, with its associated qualities, predominates during two of these zones— one during the day and one during the night. Contemporary science is beginning to corroborate much of what the ancients already knew about how aligning our routines with the dosha clock is integral to a balanced state of health. The circadian cycle that's described by the dosha clock is extremely important when it comes to strengthening our digestion, immune system, and potential for longevity—and observing the dosha clock with regularity can lead to optimal sleep hygiene.[18]

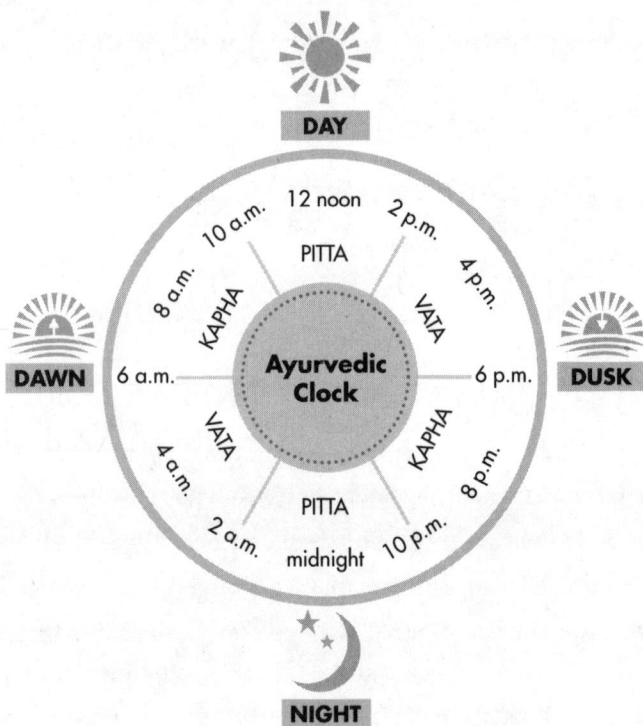

You can use the description of the dosha clock below to recognize how the body follows natural cycles—and to start placing your body at the very center of your day.

6 to 10 a.m.

This time of day is dominated by Kapha energy, associated with the elements of water and earth and their qualities. It's cool (and usually damp) outside, and nature is slowly waking up. During this period, the body can feel dull and heavy. You may feel slightly congested. Your digestion is still in the process of waking up and may need additional support to function. Many of our patients notice that if they sleep past 6 a.m., moving further into Kapha time, they actually end up feeling more sluggish and tired. That's why it's advised to wake up around 6; if you wake up later, you can kick-start your body into motion with some exercise as movement will lighten and invigorate the heavy, slow qualities of Kapha. Unless you have a job that requires physical exertion and thus a larger a.m. meal, the best way to start the day is with a light breakfast to balance the heaviness of Kapha time.

10 a.m. to 2 p.m.

As the Kapha time of day wanes, we move into the Pitta hours, associated with fire and water qualities. This is the time when the sun is highest in the sky, and when the digestive system is at its most active. It's ideal to eat your biggest meal of the day during this period, as the highest levels of hydrochloric acid secretion in the stomach are present at this time, while the body prepares to digest. If you don't eat, you may feel "hangry," the combination of hungry and angry that comes from not feeding the fire. The mind is also most focused, so Pitta time is ideal for bringing your attention to any activities that require mental agility and critical thinking. This is not the time to go out and do your most intense exercise, however, as this can cause Pitta to get out of balance and potentially affect how you sleep that night.

2 to 6 p.m.

During this time, Vata qualities dominate. Vata, representing the elements of space and air, brings creativity and inspiration to our activities. However, because Vata tends to be in motion, if you didn't eat a proper lunch or get enough fluids, you might feel tired and fatigued. If you did a lot of mental activity earlier, you may have difficulty focusing during this time. The light and quick energy of Vata can turn on a dime into anxiety and instability, so it's not uncommon for people to take a coffee break or reach for an afternoon snack. Before you get to Vata time, it's a good idea to have already eaten a grounding, fulfilling meal. You might still find that you need to rest between different activities during this period. Overall, this is a great opportunity to make art, write, take a walk, or do any other creative activity that captures the inspiring energy of Vata.

Overall, you'll want to calm that energy that has accumulated over the day with a meditation or breathing practice; otherwise, you'll take the excess Vata into your sleeping hours. It's also smart to eat your final meal of the day by the end of this window, as you are now transitioning back to Kapha time.

6 to 10 p.m.

Now, we head into the evening hours, making the switch back to Kapha. This is when the body starts to feel duller and heavier, in preparation for sunset and sleep. Digestion is already slowing, so consuming anything (especially heavy foods) in this window isn't ideal. It's best to focus on light work and light exercise, and embrace the calming nature of Kapha, so that by the end of this period, your body and mind feel ready for sleep. This is not the time to energize yourself with stimulating exercise or activities as this will interfere with the natural urge to sleep.

10 p.m. to 2 a.m.

Here, we circle back to Pitta. The body is active, but not in the same way it was during the day. A lot of our patients tell us they get a second wind around this time and actually enjoy working. However, Pitta energy should now be focused inward for tissue healing, cellular metabolism, and detoxification. This is an important period for deeper sleep cycles, which are necessary in order to cleanse the brain and body. Daytime Pitta energy was mainly focused on digestion, whereas nighttime Pitta slows down digestion of food as the liver does its thing and cellular digestion and metabolism kick in. During these hours, your body is transforming nutrients into the tissues, hormones, and enzymes that are necessary for your waking functions. Again, we have a lot of clients who enjoy working or socializing into the wee hours, when they say they feel more alert. They've caught the crest of the Pitta wave and want to ride it to the end, but in the long run, this detracts from the body's need to use Pitta energy for cell rejuvenation and detoxification. Also, if you stay awake during this pivotal time, you run the risk of feeling hungry and eating late in the night—disrupting your digestion and sleep even further.

2 to 6 a.m.

This is the Vata time of night, when we experience less deep sleep and more dream sleep. In fact, sleep science has confirmed that, although we cycle through all stages of sleep during the night, we spend more time in REM sleep and dreaming during this Vata period. Dreams can be much more vivid during this time. Quite often, you may find yourself stirred awake. Instead of feeling groggy (a quality dominated by Kapha), you're likely to feel light and alert (a quality dominated by Vata). Many people with insomnia find their minds racing with thoughts if they wake up during this time—or they might wake up while in the midst of a dream. This should come as no surprise, since Vata creates a highly active mind. You can use the end of the Vata time to help you wake up. It's actually a lot easier to wake up before 6 a.m., after which time Kapha dominates again. This is a great time to meditate or journal as you center and ground yourself for the day or release any thoughts that have accumulated through the night. You can then begin your Kapha balancing routine to get your day started.

Many of our clients have found that sticking as close to the daily rhythms of the dosha clock as possible helps them feel their best and accomplish their goals more effectively. Unfortunately, we have a tendency to disobey our body's natural impulses—for example, we have a lot of patients who tell us they get tired at 9 p.m. but it's too early to sleep, so they force themselves to stay up for a few hours. People feel that this is the only time they have for themselves; they need to "wind down" or catch up on bills, cleaning, etc.

However, as Ayurveda recognizes, and as we've discussed in the context of circadian rhythms, the more we're out of sync with our biological cycles, the more we increase our risk of both physical and mental health issues. Specific functions occur during specific times of the night and in different sleep stages. If we're awake when we should be asleep, we're missing out on our opportunity to optimize our body's functions during those times. And if we're forcing activities upon the body when the lotus is in the process of closing, this can result in a lot of health issues. For example, since digestion is not optimized at night, it's harder to digest food, and as we are typically inactive, food can be stored as excess sugar or fat. This also increases our risk of acid reflux, snoring, and sleep apnea, all of which negatively affect the quality of our sleep.

Dr. Sheila has been seeing a patient with sleep issues for several years in her primary care practice. Grace is a seventy-five-year-old woman who had several medical conditions when they first met, including prediabetes and obesity. She wanted to treat her conditions as naturally as possible using lifestyle management and had seen a functional-medicine provider for guidance. Grace implemented many healthy changes, such as regular physical activity, meditation, eating an anti-inflammatory diet, and taking anti-inflammatory supplements for a short while. She was able to get her blood sugar under control with these changes but found it challenging to lose weight.

After a few years, it was noted in routine labs that Grace's liver tests were slightly elevated, so she had a workup that included an ultrasound of her liver. A subsequent MRI showed significant fatty liver changes. Grace didn't drink alcohol or take medications that would cause this, and her "bad" cholesterol was normal, although her "good" cholesterol was low. Upon further questioning, it turned out that while she was doing and eating the right things, she was eating late due to her long work hours, and not going to sleep until 1–2 a.m. She woke up at 7 a.m. feeling rested but became tired in the middle of the day. Dr. Sheila strongly recommended that Grace change the timing of her last meal and go to sleep by 10–11 p.m. Despite her other healthy efforts, Grace found it challenging to make these changes. Her liver tests eventually normalized, but she continues to show fatty liver on imaging tests, and she still finds it challenging to lose weight.

This story highlights what some studies have shown regarding the effects of sleep disturbances (in this case, sleeping late and less than the ideal number of hours) on various hormones and metabolic pathways that control weight, cholesterol metabolism, and liver functions, especially as we age.[19] Although Grace was doing everything else correctly, it's likely that the circadian disruption decreased her capacity to experience optimal health. This aligns with the Ayurvedic perspective that she was missing key detoxification and metabolism times by missing out on the functions of Pitta during the hours of 10 p.m. and 2 a.m.

Since we know it can be challenging to change long-established sleep patterns, one way to reboot and rebuild a daily schedule is to undergo a period of Ayurvedic detoxification, or *panchakarma*. When there is a lot of built-up toxicity in your physiology, it can be hard to rebalance, even when you're doing "all the right things." If this sounds familiar to you, perhaps an Ayurvedic detox is in order.

PANCHAKARMA PERKS: REFRESH YOUR BODY AND MIND

Overall, the dosha clock gives us a precise picture of what our body is doing related to all these periods and cycles—and what we can do to support our body's functions. During various seasons, one or the other of the doshas' qualities will increase and can lead to imbalances later, so seasonal cleanses are often recommended in Ayurveda. This can help reboot the system and reconnect us to our natural sleep rhythms.

Vata generally tends to dominate from the early autumn through early winter, Pitta from late spring to late summer, and Kapha from late winter to early spring. During their respective season, as with their time of the day, the dosha accumulates. Therefore, Ayurveda generally advises that a Vata cleanse occur around the summer and winter solstices, a Pitta cleanse around fall equinox, and a Kapha cleanse around spring equinox.

Of course, this example is applicable to a typical four-season climate, but it's important to remember that seasons vary across the globe. Some places have six seasons, some have four, some have two, and others remain pretty much the same throughout the year. Climate change has also shifted our expectations of how the seasons should look and feel. In addition, even though a dosha-specific cleanse at each seasonal transition is always a good idea, it may be preferable to base your cleanse on your own specific needs or dosha aggravations. You can work directly with a trained Ayurvedic practitioner to get a sense of how you can sync with the seasons.

Many of our clients find that if they've been off balance with their sleep schedule, panchakarma is a good way to reset an off-kilter circadian rhythm. *Panchakarma* refers to a seasonal Ayurvedic cleanse and translates to "five actions," which encompass five traditional techniques or methods that help to regulate our doshic balance. Today, however, these methods may not all be used at once during a seasonal cleanse.

Dr. Suhas has a memorable case of working with a fifty-two-year-old Japanese stockbroker. Kenji lived in Tokyo but dialed in to New York every night as soon as the market opened. With the fourteen-hour time difference, he was talking to New York late at night and was dead tired by the time he began trading in Japan. Kenji had been doing all this for close to a decade and was at the apex of his career, but his health was failing. He was diagnosed with metabolic syndrome (a condition that increases one's risk of diabetes, stroke, and heart disease) and extreme insomnia. Despite his fatigue, he was unable to sleep, and his nervous system was in a continuously jittery state. Even when he closed his eyes, his eyelids flickered—an expression of Vata imbalance.

After Kenji made a decision that lost one of his clients several million dollars, he knew he needed to make a change, so he checked into Dr. Suhas's clinic for fourteen days of panchakarma. He shared that he was unable to focus, and he was anxious and depressed. He feared that he'd never be functional again. Kenji had been given sleeping pills by his doctor, but he reported that they'd actually worsened his symptoms of daytime fatigue and hadn't really helped him to sleep.

His protocol of Ayurvedic treatments included *shirodhara*, which entails a slow, steady, rhythmic stream of special Ayurvedic herbs and oils poured over the forehead to calm the nervous system and balance the doshas. (In fact, there are studies that confirm the benefits of shirodhara on sleep.)[20] On the first day of his program during this treatment, something amazing happened: Kenji fell into a deep sleep that left him feeling more restored than he had been in a long time.

On the second day, Kenji didn't come to the afternoon meal, which made staff members at the clinic begin to worry. It wasn't until several hours later that he finally emerged from his room. As it turned out, Kenji had gone straight to his room after the shirodhara treatment and had fallen asleep. Over the next two weeks of his treatment, he regularly slept for six or seven hours every night. Kenji also attended regular counseling sessions, where Dr. Suhas helped him determine the lifestyle measures he needed to put in place to keep his frazzled nervous system from going over the edge.

Dr. Suhas informed Kenji that because his was a chronic imbalance—especially since he also traveled to New York fifteen to twenty times a year—he'd have to do a detox every three months, given the disruption that was occurring in his body on a cellular level. He'd spent too much time in unnatural settings and had been confusing every cell of his body for so long that they had forgotten what to do and when. In his case, he needed to do at least two long cleanses (fourteen days) in the fall and spring and two shorter cleanses (seven days) in the winter and summer to resync with his circadian rhythm.

Kenji worked with Dr. Suhas for a full year and was very happy with the results. His depression subsided, his energy returned, and his severe cognitive decline improved. He developed a consistent meditation practice and improved his nutritional habits between cleanses. Incredibly, despite all the days he took off to commit to the detox sessions, Kenji's business was more successful and abundant than ever before. His limiting belief that his office wouldn't be able to function without him had been wrong all along. Unsurprisingly, his chronic insomnia, which had been plaguing his life for close to ten years, was having an effect on his functioning and productivity. It took a year of cleanses and changes to his lifestyle to reset his system.

Stories like Kenji's are good reminders that living in accordance with the laws of nature can help us bask in the afterglow of awakened sleep, which touches every aspect of our lives. Ideally, you'll be able to catch imbalances before they become extreme and realign with your natural rhythms and sleep cycle to function at your best in body, mind, and spirit.

ASSESSMENT: YOUR DOSHA CLOCK—
TIME YOUR PERFECT DAY

Use the dosha clock below to methodically go through your own typical schedule. Note the following:

1. What are you usually doing during the classic dosha time periods?
2. Do your activities and mental states correspond to the ideal activities and mental states that are dictated by the dosha clock? If not, can you take stock of how this might be taking you out of sync with your natural rhythms?
3. What season of life are you in (childhood/Kapha, adulthood/Pitta, or mature years/Vata), and how is this affecting your dosha balance?

4. Can you identify two to three small changes to aid in greater balance throughout your day? Write them down below:

    o _____

    o _____

    o _____

REFLECTIONS

1. Would you consider yourself a morning bird, night owl, or something else altogether?
   a. What habits in your life have contributed to your self-ascribed chronotype?
   b. Has it always been this way, or have your life circumstances changed your sleep schedule (and times of most alertness during the day) over time?
2. Note what the seasons are like in the area where you live. What are the changes you notice with respect to your own sleep cycle as the seasons transition?
3. How would you like to try balancing your life with solar, lunar, and seasonal cycles?

List any takeaways from this chapter that you'd like to incorporate into your own sleep-hygiene routine:

_____

_____

_____

_____

_____

CHAPTER 4

WHAT HAPPENS WHEN SLEEP TAKES A BACK SEAT?

Happiness, misery, nourishment, emaciation,
strength, weakness, virility, sterility, knowledge,
ignorance, life and death—all these occur
depending on the proper or improper sleep.

—*Charaka Samhita*, Sutrasthana 21/36

ACCORDING TO THE *CHARAKA SAMHITA*, YOUR LIFE AND DEATH depend upon the quality of your sleep. It might sound like an exaggeration, but it isn't. As the ancients knew, and as we've already emphasized throughout the last few chapters, there is no single part of us that isn't affected by our sleep.

Unfortunately, the disruption of healthy sleep patterns has been linked to far more than early-morning crankiness. Among the ramifications of poor sleep, you can count a range of chronic disorders that affect our physical, mental/emotional, and spiritual health. Poor sleep increases our risk of obesity, poor digestion, hypertension, heart disease, diabetes, dementia, cancer, and mortality. Not to mention, mental health disorders are at an all-time high, and science continues to reveal a growing awareness that sleep problems directly contribute to depression, anxiety, and suicidal ideation.

These are the side effects of poor-quality shut-eye, and the problem is only expected to worsen over the coming years, especially with environmental determinants like light pollution and modern lifestyles affecting our daily rhythms.

Of course, the consequences of poor sleep go well beyond the physiological and psychological effects and may have consequences that modern science isn't aware of yet. When we aren't getting deep, restorative sleep, we are missing out on one of the primary ways to tap into the power of consciousness. It's during sleep that we can access our full potential for repairing the daily wear and tear and rejuvenating our minds after all the activities and thoughts associated with our day-to-day. In other words, health and healing are the outcome of moving into a more expanded consciousness, and we have the opportunity to do that every night! So, in order to lead a healthy and happy life, it's not enough to eat well or exercise on a daily basis; we would venture to say that, if you're not actively prioritizing sleep, you are compromising your overall health—regardless of how much else you're doing to care for it.

Throughout this chapter, we'll share some of the impacts of sleeplessness and poor sleep. This is not meant to be an all-inclusive list of the effects of poor sleep but to highlight what has been observed for thousands of years: We don't experience optimal well-being in body, mind, and spirit without healthy sleep. The purpose of sharing all this isn't to scare you but to drive home the fact that sleep is more important than we have given it credit for in our modern world. We understand that knowledge is key, so understanding what happens when we don't sleep will empower you with everything you need to make long-term, sustainable change possible.

SLEEP, BODY, AND BRAIN: A JOYFUL, ENERGETIC BODY

When we don't get enough or quality sleep, we run the risk of many physical disorders, including early mortality. A recent study found that younger people who practiced good sleep hygiene were a lot less likely to die at an early age.[1] And a 2017 review of the consequences of sleep disruption confirms that poor sleep is associated with many short- and long-term health consequences.[2] Short-term effects include increased activity of the sympathetic nervous system (fight-or-flight physiology), metabolic effects, and pro-inflammatory responses, among others. This results in an increased risk of hypertension, dyslipidemia, cardiovascular disease, weight-related issues, metabolic syndrome, type 2 diabetes mellitus, colorectal cancer, and all-cause mortality in some groups in the long term. The pro-inflammatory effect is worrisome because chronic inflammation (long-term inflammation that can last for months or years) has been linked not only to a higher risk of diabetes and heart disease but also to arthritis, cancer, and dementia, among other health conditions.[3] Ultimately, keeping the doshas balanced and creating healthy sleep involves reducing chronic inflammation through the lifestyle practices discussed in this book.

Inflammation (both acute and chronic) can affect areas of the brain associated with sleep and interfere with the body's sleep/wake cycle. To make matters worse, poor sleep can then exacerbate inflammation.[4] We can end up in several vicious cycles when it comes to inflammation. For example, when inflammation is associated with pain conditions and is not brought under control, the pain can further disrupt sleep.

When it comes to the brain, there's a growing body of research connecting a lack of quality sleep with poor cognitive function, cognitive decline, and dementia in old age.[5] Many of our older patients often tell us, "I don't care if I'm frail when I'm older—I just don't want to lose my mental faculties." This is why we spend a large part of each patient visit asking about sleep, regardless of the chief complaint. We emphasize the importance of creating a lifestyle and a set of habits that prioritize our sleep—well before we hit the Vata, or old age phase of life.

How does Ayurveda make sense of the research linking poor sleep with poor brain health? Before research described this association, Ayurveda made the connection. According to Ayurveda, there are seven primary tissues in the human body. The first is called *rasa*, and it refers to the clear part of the blood, loosely translated as "serum" or "plasma" in Western medicine. Rasa is our body's clear fluids and also includes lymph and interstitial fluid—the fluid that leaks from the blood vessels and into the space between cells due to osmotic pressure. However, any lost fluid needs to ultimately be brought back into our circulatory system in order to be healthy; if that rasa is lost, it leads to what's known as lymphatic stagnation, which can create a sense of puffiness, bloating, and heaviness.

Lymphatic stagnation is similar to having a pile of unwashed linens—it's only by recirculating that fluid in our blood that we can be healthy. In addition, when we bring fluid and waste from the intracellular space into lymphatic vessels and to lymph nodes, we are informing our immune system and allowing it to function more effectively. Through the flow of lymph, we are directing waste back to the blood to be removed. Ayurveda considers this waste toxicity, or ama, as it has the potential to cause disease. So, clearing the body of toxins through the flow of rasa is essential for health. Our rasa gives us a close-up of our state of health. When Ayurvedic doctors observe patients' rasa, they determine whether that person is in good health. Improving the quality of rasa is a practice known as *rasayana*, which is performed through diet, massage, herbs, yoga, and other remedies that direct the lymph back into circulation.

How does this relate to sleep and brain health? Well, there are no lymph vessels in the brain to clean out metabolic waste and soluble proteins; instead, the recently identified glymphatic system, which is a network of channels between cells in the brain, does the work of cleansing and detoxifying this important region of the body. And that cleansing and detoxifying activity in the brain is most prominent at night, during our deep-sleep cycles. Many scientists speculate that if our deep-sleep cycles are disrupted, it can lead to a toxic accumulation of protein sediments in the brain— which may result in Alzheimer's disease and other forms of dementia, as well as other cognitive disorders. There are studies that show that a lack of deep sleep (slow-wave sleep) can increase the risk of dementia but that this is a risk factor that can be modified.[6] From an Ayurvedic perspective, this involves optimizing sleep, especially during those valuable Pitta hours (10 p.m. to 2 a.m.).

Essentially, if you're not sleeping well, your rasa will be compromised, and your body's ability to cleanse and detoxify your brain and body will also be compromised, setting you up for chronic illness. Every time you "lose" sleep, keep erratic hours, or move through different time zones, you affect the quality of your rasa. For this reason, Ayurveda places a lot of value on massage (which helps move lymph to the lymph nodes for cleansing) and other forms of rasayana. In Ayurvedic medicine, massage is considered medical treatment and is typically part of an Ayurvedic treatment plan, whether it's done by practitioners or as part of a daily routine of self-massage.

SLEEP AND YOUR MIND: REFLECTIVE AND ALERT

Without restorative sleep, our mind is not clear, we can't focus, and we wake up on the proverbial wrong side of the bed, in the sense that we don't feel our natural state of joy upon rising in the morning. Indeed, science has confirmed that poor sleep can lead to an increased risk of depression and anxiety symptoms, and that improved sleep quality has the capacity to reduce these symptoms.

So, apart from making us feel tired and foggy, poor sleep affects our emotions and how we end up responding (or reacting) to the world around us. Getting insufficient or poor sleep can result in compromised concentration, spaciness, irritability, and a general feeling of wanting to crawl back under the covers rather than face the world. You are less likely to offer a sympathetic ear or heartfelt words of wisdom and connection to someone who really needs it if you're struggling with insomnia and fatigue. An unbalanced emotional state ends up affecting your relationships, work and career, and all aspects of life. In fact, a large meta-analysis confirmed a link between sleep loss, negative mood, and affective functioning (social and emotional functioning), so it's vital for our mental and emotional health to pay attention to our sleep.[7]

With the 24/7 nature of the news and social media, our subjective quality of sleep has a lot to do with the toxicity that we are exposed to. According to an article in *The Atlantic*,[8] a "bad" mood is often the most important determinant in someone's online etiquette. Not surprisingly, internet trolls are most active late at night and least active in the early morning. Most of us are also aware of the adage "Let me sleep on it," which suggests that we innately understand good decisions are made when we give ourselves time to rest and digest the day. Too many bad, impulse-driven decisions are made late at night, sometimes in the throes of an "I can't sleep" moment. And this is only amplified when we are chronically sleep-deprived.

When we experience acute emotional stress, we can initiate an acute inflammatory response, which has a detrimental effect on sleep. An emotional factor might be an argument, loss of a job, driving in traffic day after day, or any stressful life situation. Regardless of the cause, all these circumstances can lead to an acute inflammatory cytokine release in the body, which happens when the immune system responds in hyperdrive to the stressor. Cytokines are tiny proteins that signal the immune system to do its job. However, these proteins have been found to interfere with sleep duration and depth. And when we experience chronic stress, this can lead to chronic sleep disruption. This can then lead to another one of those vicious cycles. Insomnia has been shown to increase the risk of depression and anxiety, and feelings of depression and anxiety can further interfere with sleep.

From an Ayurvedic perspective, we can have optimal awakened sleep only if we regulate our emotions and keep our minds stable and focused, as we will take any unresolved mental turbulence into the night with us. And if we have turbulent, nonrestful sleep, we perpetuate imbalances in the mind. We'll dive deeper into the concept of the mind later, but suffice it to say that Ayurveda deeply recognizes the connection of sleep to mental and emotional health.

Do We Really Need Eight Hours of Sleep?

We've been taught that we need eight hours of sleep in order for our body to function at its optimal level. However, from a medical perspective, this isn't entirely true. The amount of sleep we need varies based on our age. Ayurveda is clear that lack of sleep can interfere with our mood and general vitality and that it affects us across all our life stages.

As we learned earlier, classical Ayurvedic texts suggest that there are three general life stages: youth (characterized by Kapha dominance), middle age (characterized by Pitta dominance), and old age (characterized by Vata dominance). High-quality sleep has been shown to be important in all stages of life. Although childhood is characterized by increased Kapha energy, which allows us to sleep more soundly, sleep issues can begin in childhood. Children are also susceptible to the factors that disrupt sleep in our modern world, and sleep disorders can affect up to 30 percent of children and cause significant health issues. During the Pitta time of life, adults often experience the effects of stress, overwork, and overactivity, which all disrupt sleep and affect all areas of life. And during the Vata phase of life, older people notice a reduction in the quantity and quality of their sleep, with up to 50 percent of older adults complaining about sleep issues, as the normal homeostatic mechanisms that allow us to sleep become less efficient.

But how much sleep is enough? In general, we know that infants require a great deal more sleep than young children. From young adulthood to our elderly years, the amount of sleep that's advised tends to be the same. In fact, chronic health issues tend to be higher among people who sleep less than six hours or more than nine hours, which suggests there's a generally optimal amount of sleep that people need. However, as we explore the possibility of awakened sleep, the rule of thumb that says eight hours of sleep is best starts to wobble.

Getting about seven hours of sleep can be enough to increase the quality of your life and sharpen the functions of your mind and body. But modern science is finding that quality, timing, and regularity are more important than quantity alone. One person can have an excellent period of sleep in a consistent three- to four-hour spurt each night while another could get the requisite eight hours and still feel exhausted by the time their alarm jolts them awake. It has been shown that there is a fine balance between too little and too much sleep for most people. There is an association between cognitive decline and sleeping less than five hours or more than ten hours per night. This is also in alignment with the Ayurvedic concept of balance—we don't function optimally with too little, or too much, sleep.[9]

In Ayurveda, there are stories of enlightened yogis and sages who embodied the concept of awakened sleep—many needing only a few hours of sleep yet maintaining excellent health. Although these stories may seem far-fetched or out of reach for most of us, we all have the potential to achieve what these other humans have. We will explore some of the practices that allowed these adepts to maximize their potential during sleep. In general, according to Ayurveda, the ideal sleep period is between sunset and sunrise, and sleeping between 10 p.m. and 4 a.m. is ideal for the body's systems.

With the addition of tools that offer the experience of awakened sleep, you might discover you can sleep more efficiently—just as you may have discovered that it's possible to do less and achieve more when you incorporate meditation into your life. You've probably experienced this form of "bending time" at some point or another. Perhaps you had nights when you didn't sleep for too long, but you felt enlivened, energetic, and happy. It's possible to take these isolated incidents and turn them into your new normal, whether you get eight hours of sleep or not.

SLEEP AND SPIRIT: A LOVING, COMPASSIONATE HEART

Aside from the fact that poor sleep creates a massive strain on our bodies and minds, too many people are living out the effects of poor sleep on the spirit—in the form of discontentment in relationships, lack of purpose or meaning, as well as a general feeling of disconnection.

When we feel separate from everything around us, this leads to a feeling of isolation and loneliness. In fact, the 2023 US Surgeon General Advisory has deemed that we have a current epidemic of loneliness that constitutes a public health crisis. Interestingly, one study recently linked better sleep health with lower emotional and social loneliness scores.[10] This may also, in part, explain the increase in depressive symptoms when we don't sleep. When we consider the concept of connecting to spirit (or consciousness) during sleep as Vedic science describes, we can actually use sleep to cultivate a sense of oneness and connectedness to everything around us, as we discuss further in the next section. Through awakened sleep practices, we can feel less lonely, connect to meaning, and feel more at peace.

One of the best ways to experience a sense of connectedness is to immerse ourselves in nature. When we talk to our patients, it's clear that all of them want a deeper connection to their spirituality, but they don't know how to expand this area of life outside of organized religion. More studies are being dedicated to understanding this realm of our experience, which does not necessarily have to mean an affiliation with any particular religion. Although there is much debate, it is clear that, as human beings, we all have spiritual experiences, and that there are distinct qualities of consciousness we engage with via spiritual practices. These qualities include joy/bliss, compassion, equanimity, love, and transcendence. Thankfully, there are many ways to experience these qualities of spirit or consciousness.

As many of our patients have shared, getting back to our nature and rebalancing our lives can prove to be difficult, especially in our modern world full of technology and artificial "fixes" that are meant to keep us in a constant state of busyness and productivity. In some ways, while technology has made our lives much easier and more convenient, it has also resulted in a disconnection from our nature via the sleep/wake cycle, which is such a critical component of our spiritual health.

One of the major keys to reconnecting with our true nature is unplugging and spending time with Mother Nature. One of Dr. Sheila's patients, Bruno, was deeply influenced by something she once told him: "You need to touch the Earth in order to find balance." Bruno took her words quite literally, and they changed his life. Bruno was living in Brazil and had a typical hectic life. He felt disconnected from himself, but he wistfully remembered a time when he had more of a lightness of being. He wasn't sleeping, wasn't feeling joyful, and had several physical issues at play. He took a leap of faith and decided to go on a three-month sabbatical and immerse himself in the jungles of the Amazon. During this time, he wasn't driving or using his phone or computer. It was just Bruno, his dog, and his yoga practice—in the thick of the rainforest.

Many months later, he shared how much this period of time had transformed him. "I hadn't realized that I was always dealing with a low-key anxiety that ruled my entire life—not until I took the time to be with myself, the Earth, the bird sounds, and this feeling that the tempo of life was completely different from the artificial one I'd taken on. I began to sleep better than I had in years, my mood improved, and I felt energized, like I was young again," said Bruno, who looked about ten years younger when Dr. Sheila saw him again. At a time when most people fear that letting go of technology will feel disconnecting, Bruno actually felt more of a connection through nature.

Often, we've found that certain suggestions will hit our individual patients in a very specific way and take them on their own path to awakened sleep. This usually means reconnecting to a sense of wonder and awe, be it through nature, a creative endeavor, or connecting to a community of like-minded people who help uplift our spirit. As someone who'd always loved the outdoors, Bruno took Dr. Sheila's suggestion as an opportunity to return to that original love, which helped him to rebuild a connection with his spirit—and to get the restorative sleep he'd felt deprived of for years.

THE ORIGINAL BIOHACK

In many ways, Ayurveda is the original biohacking methodology, because it enables us to use a variety of interventions to connect us to a deeper understanding of who we are. It just requires us to begin to connect within and to how we feel *qualitatively*, not *quantitatively*. In other words, it requires us to connect to our subjective experience for answers.

Of course, we want to be very mindful here as we are not suggesting that technology is the enemy. Indeed, there are many sleep-tracking apps and other forms of technology that our patients have turned to on their quest for awakened sleep. Advances in sleep technology have given rise to a fascinating array of tools that help decode our nightly routines. Today, you can find everything from wearables, patches, headbands, and wrist devices to systems that use biofeedback, audio cues, and visualizations to shed light on your sleep patterns. These innovations offer fresh insights into how you rest and provide new ways to improve your sleep quality. (For more details on these evolving technologies, feel free to explore our website, www.awakenedsleep.net.)

It can be helpful to collect objective data about sleep, and our tech is improving by the hour. A recent study showed that most wearable digital devices provide fairly accurate information; at the same time, it's a good idea to question our dependency on technology.[11] We've both had patients who feel enriched by sleep apps, but we've also had those whose perception of their own health was negatively affected after introducing the apps into their life. For example, some of our clients have tracked their sleep with the assumption that they're sleeping well—only to see the "data" and feel crushed by what appears to be a poor sleep pattern. This can be especially unhelpful for someone with a Vata imbalance who might already be experiencing anxiety in this domain of their life. More objective information to focus on isn't always better. One of the most important aspects of Ayurvedic and Vedic wisdom is its emphasis on helping us to gain interoceptive (that is, information based on internal stimuli) awareness of ourselves. The process of coming to know ourselves, and maintaining an inner and outer ecosystem that helps us preserve balance, is one of the deep gifts of awakened sleep.

When we understand ourselves in the context of nature, we know ourselves at a deeper level than objective data allows for. Just like everything in nature, we experience different seasons of life, in which various doshas dominate. As you've learned already, during a particular dosha season, we experience more of the qualities of that dosha. We have different physical and emotional needs as we transition from childhood to adulthood during puberty; similarly, we need to recognize shifts in our physiology as we age. If we have irregular schedules, travel frequently, don't hydrate, and overstimulate all of our senses, we are more likely to experience Vata imbalances, especially as we enter the Vata time of life (after age fifty to sixty). This shows up as many of the typical health conditions we see with aging, such as constipation, insomnia, dryness, diminished brain health, and other neurological conditions.

From an Ayurvedic perspective, rasa/lymph is associated with Kapha dosha, which is the aspect of our physiology that is watery and lubricating and is abundant in childhood (the Kapha time of life) but decreases as we age; it regulates all the "fountains" in our body, providing us with "grease" or liquid that keeps us from drying out. For patients at a Vata age who also have a Vata-aggravating lifestyle, matters can worsen if they're not paying enough attention to their sleep. We see some of our older patients attempting to work, play, and exercise in the same ways they did decades prior. But you can't live the same way at age seventy-five that you did at thirty-five and stay in balance; there are natural effects of aging that don't necessarily show up as disease but rather as slowing down and needing more time for recovery.

Take the example of June, a sixty-year-old woman who came to us with complaints about her ability to sleep. As we inquired about her daily habits, we learned that her life is packed to the brim with activities. June also shared that she tries to stay active by playing sports several hours a day, even when her body is shouting at her to stop. With that combination of physical and mental exertion, it was little wonder that her sleep was suffering. Although June can't fit everything into her busy schedule and often goes to sleep with her stomach in knots over everything on her growing to-do list, she insisted, "I can't possibly slow down! I have four years until I retire, and I'm trying to knock out several goals all at once."

This is a common complaint we hear from patients, many of whom are just around the corner from retirement age. However, we always share with them that the quality of their time *right now* matters. June's high-intensity schedule is interfering with her ability to get the most out of her sleep. And, at this age, she needs to do whatever she can to manage that high-strung Vata energy. Often, we find that our patients worry about slowing down. They worry that if they try to relax now, they'll simply wither into old age and a sedentary life. But overactivity can be enough to wipe out an otherwise strong and active person in their Vata years. We always explain to patients that slowing down to enjoy life and prioritize sleep hygiene enables us to engage with greater self-care and appreciation of the present moment, which enhances both quality and quantity of life.

What many people at the Vata stage often find is that, by the time they're ready to retire, a lifetime of unhelpful habits that have impinged upon their quality of sleep has caught up to them. Although many older people are living to a later and later age, they're also carrying with them chronic health issues that hamper their ability to truly enjoy the time they have. You're probably familiar with the idea of lifespan, which is the number of years we live. But we now need to consider our *health span* as well. This refers to our number of healthy years free from disease. What's the point of having a long lifespan if our health span could end up being so much shorter? This is where the power of awakened sleep comes in. Not only does it expand our health span—it also makes it such that we can truly soak up the goodness life has to offer. As in so many other of the cases we've explored throughout this book, the trick to your lifespan—and your health span—can often be traced back to supporting natural sleep.

Sex and Sleep—Find Your Sweet Spot

Sexual activity is a natural and essential part of life, and from an Ayurvedic standpoint, it can contribute positively to our overall well-being and even enhance sleep. The key is balance. *Shukra* (a Sanskrit word that refers to our reproductive system and sexual essence and energy), when treated with respect and care, replenishes vitality, nourishes the body, and can improve longevity. However, like all aspects of life, it must be approached mindfully to avoid disrupting our sleep.

The desire for sex is not something that should be suppressed, nor should it be overindulged. Ayurveda views it as a natural urge (vega) that, when engaged in healthily, can foster emotional connection, deepen intimacy with one's partner, and create a sense of warmth that aids in restful sleep. After sexual activity, it's recommended to relieve the body by using the restroom and, if possible, taking a warm shower to cleanse and calm oneself.

The timing of sexual activity is crucial. Ayurveda advises against engaging in sex immediately after meals as digestion takes precedence at that time. It is also best avoided during times of illness, menstruation, or during the first and third trimesters of pregnancy as these can be times of heightened sensitivity or energy depletion. If possible, a warm cup of milk can help replenish energy post activity, especially in the context of shukra replenishment.

Overall, it's a good idea to approach sexual activity by infusing it with a wholesome quality. In other words, the experience should be mindful, not something driven solely by raw desire or emotional imbalance. Emotional connection with a healthy partner promotes a sense of harmony within, enhancing the quality of sleep rather than disturbing it. Engaging in sex during emotional or physical conflict, or when feeling mentally unsettled, can lead to overstimulation and imbalances that leak into our slumber.

In Ayurveda, the evening is considered a *tamasic* period, or a time when the mind tends to become clouded, and can give way to habitual tendencies, such as indulging in obsessive sexual thoughts or hedonistic pleasures. If these desires become overwhelming, they can lead to a sense of disequilibrium that you take into your sleep. However, if you are engaging in healthy sexual activity with a supportive, balanced partner, and it's done mindfully, it shouldn't block your ability for awakened sleep. Healthy sexual energy, when properly channeled, can align with restful sleep, not hinder it.

Of course, during life phases like perimenopause and menopause, many women experience both sleep issues and a drop in libido due to hormonal shifts. Ayurveda suggests addressing this imbalance by nourishing the body with grounding foods like ghee and root vegetables, and supporting vitality with adaptogens such as ashwagandha. Self-care practices like meditation and warm-oil massage can calm the nervous system, improve circulation, and restore energy, potentially enhancing both sexual desire and sleep quality.

Ultimately, sex is a healthy part of life, but it must be integrated into your routine with mindfulness and respect for your body's rhythms. Balance, emotional connection, and timing are essential in ensuring that sex enhances your ability to fall into a restful, rejuvenating sleep. When practiced mindfully, it becomes a tool for longevity, vitality, and overall well-being.

CHANGE YOUR HABITS; CHANGE YOUR LIFE

The most important thing to remember is that lifestyle changes that result in better sleep can be as simple as shifting one or two aspects of your daily routine. Minor tweaks can help support every aspect of your well-being and lead to awakened sleep.

The physical, mental/emotional, and spiritual effects of a hectic lifestyle and poor sleep are evident in a patient that Dr. Suhas recently worked with. Bao, a thirty-four-year-old Singaporean man who had moved to San Francisco and was working in IT, had a team that was composed of people who spanned the globe—from Hong Kong to Taiwan to the US. One of Bao's projects was especially demanding; on top of his regular day job, he was up every night from 7:30 p.m. to 1:30 a.m. to work with his colleagues in Asia. Both his office and home became places associated with high stress. Bao didn't know how long the project would last, only that it had come to consume his waking (and sleeping) hours.

When Bao came to Dr. Suhas, he was drinking coffee and energy drinks nonstop to power through the morning and the evening. He got about five hours of uninterrupted but erratic sleep every night—during which he was sometimes so restless that he'd wake up to watch TV or pore over a work issue he was afraid he hadn't resolved—before waking up and having to do it all over again. Sadly, many other aspects of Bao's life suffered. He had been in a long-term relationship that recently ended, in no small part due to Bao's obsessive work habits. His sex drive and self-esteem were totally diminished. It was clear from his emaciated frame, the dark circles under his eyes, his fidgety mannerisms, and the way he looked down rather than making eye contact that he was severely depressed and lonely and felt little purpose in his work. He was on the fast track to chronic disease and needed help.

Dr. Suhas gently urged Bao to talk to his boss and explain that his workload wasn't sustainable. Bao insisted that he couldn't do that; however, for three months, he agreed to work with Dr. Suhas to create a proper sleep protocol. Over time, Bao began to see things more clearly; he became willing to change his schedule so he could work only three days a week. During the rest of the week, he visited the clinic to receive *abhyanga* (Ayurvedic oil massage) and shirodhara treatments, both of which balanced the excess Vata in Bao's system. To ground and nourish his imbalanced Vata, he also needed to adjust his diet. Although Bao didn't have the bandwidth to make his own meals, he identified high-quality homemade food that was available in his area. And while Bao had a naturally rebellious disposition and had turned away from Eastern spiritual traditions at an early age, he immediately fell in love with the meditative practices he was introduced to and worked them into his routine.

After two months, Bao had created a regular daily and nightly routine. He told Dr. Suhas that he'd always felt the most depressed when he lay in bed alone, thinking of the relationship that he'd lost. But in time, he regained enough confidence and optimism to return to the dating scene. Today, he is in a happy and healthy relationship—and has taken a new job where he doesn't have to worry about talking to members of a global team at all hours of the day and night!

Bao's case was not just one of physical depletion; in truth, many of his sleep issues were rooted in mental/emotional and spiritual depletion, which were both worsened by lack of quality sleep. Today, his regular meditation practice and efforts to connect with his emotional needs have manifested in a more fruitful and meaningful life.

This is another case that illustrates how the inability to sleep well can manifest in a cascade of symptoms that feed one another in an unhealthy cycle that derails us from the train of optimal well-being. Because sleep is connected to so many self-regulatory mechanisms in the body, when we consciously take it to the next level, we can reclaim our innate ability to rest and to experience even greater levels of health.

Of course, it all comes back to our willingness: Do we want to make a change? Although Bao didn't choose to shift out of his work conditions until several months after seeing Dr. Suhas, he took several important steps that helped him regain balance in his life. However, we both routinely work with patients who are just looking for a quick fix.

"Can you give me something to help me sleep better for the next three months?" one of Dr. Suhas's patients once asked him. She explained that, while she's healthy and physically active, she'd been watching the news leading up to the 2024 presidential election very closely—which led to a tremendous sense of anxiety, anger, and unease. "I just need to take something until all of it is over!" she insisted. The problem with such an approach is this: When will "it" ever be over? Our lives are constantly filled with internal and external agitations and sources of stress. The more we choose to participate in and churn that energy, the more we encourage it. Every thought we feed affects our waking and sleeping hours.

The truth is, there is no magic pill when it comes to sleep. Creating awakened sleep is the best long-term antidote, but it requires dedication and participation. How often have we told ourselves, "I'll sleep later. *This is more important!*" But what can be more important than sleep, which is conducive to all our physiological, mental, and spiritual processes? If lack of care for our sleep—compounded by the idea that we can fix it with a remedy that could end up having long-term side effects—is an attitude we perpetuate, we'll only continue to generate the same miserable conditions we are trying to abate!

You can give time to whatever is important to you, but you don't have to make it so all-consuming that it interferes with your overall happiness and balance. Throughout the course of life, all of us will run into moments that require more of our attention than we might like. At the very least, you can "do what you have to do" during the day and treat bedtime as sacred time. All it takes for a lifetime of awakened sleep is a little curiosity and willingness to participate in your own health—every day and every night.

As a society, our lack of sleep—and our lack of deeper awareness as to how we can use sleep to access our fundamental human potential (consciousness)—is reflected in a sense of global imbalance that's evident wherever we turn. And although you've just read about the many negative health consequences of poor sleep, the benefits of sleep transcend merely getting the necessary downtime to prevent disease. This is what enables us to connect, create, and evolve as humans. As we'll discuss in Part 2, it could very well be that sleep is the answer to far more than our health and longevity.

ASSESSMENT: WHICH SLEEP HABITS WILL YOU CHOOSE?

Now that you're aware of some of the long-term effects on your physical, mental/emotional, and spiritual health when you don't sleep, let's look at some of the things that can support natural sleep and make a note of how many of them you are currently doing, or not doing. Please remember that it's never too late to change, and even adopting one or two of these habits can radically transform your sleep hygiene and affect both your lifespan and health span!

Body
- getting adequate sunlight during the day, especially morning sun
- engaging in physical movement during the day
- eating more natural, whole foods
- eating your final meal at least two hours before bedtime
- taking an evening walk or stretching in the evening
- giving yourself a gentle self-massage before bed

Mind/Emotions

- journaling
- doing emotional-release work to let go of past experiences and emotions you are holding on to
- providing yourself with calming aromatherapy in the evening
- removing the TV from the room in which you sleep
- making gratitude lists before bed

Spirit

- chanting or singing
- engaging in meditation/prayer
- connecting to nature
- practicing present-moment awareness in your daily activities
- listening to inspiring or spiritual podcasts
- calming yoga and breathwork in the evening

REFLECTIONS

1. What have you become conscious of regarding choices and habits you've cultivated around your physical, mental/emotional, and spiritual health? How do all these choices and habits ultimately affect your sleep?
2. You're beginning to learn more about how sleep influences all aspects of life. How would you describe your life right now? How would you like it to be?
3. What choices and habits would you like to change? What would you like to exchange them with? (You can look at the checklists in the Assessments section for inspiration.)
4. What excites you about the process of cultivating better sleep hygiene and experiencing awakened sleep on a more regular basis?

5. What might feel new, uncertain, or even daunting? Once you understand your behavior, it becomes so much easier to change your habits. And remember, even a simple shift can transform your sleep and your life!

List any takeaways from this chapter that you'd like to incorporate into your own sleep-hygiene routine:

_____

_____

_____

_____

_____

PART 2

SLEEP YOUR WAY TO
JOY AND VITALITY

CHAPTER 5

)) ● ((

COME TO YOUR
SENSES IN THE
SANCTUARY OF SLEEP

How blessed are some people, whose lives have no
fears, no dreads, to whom sleep is a blessing that
comes nightly, and brings nothing but sweet dreams.

—Bram Stoker

NOW THAT WE'VE EXPLORED THE IMPACT SLEEP HAS ON ALL DIMEN-
sions of our health and well-being, we're ready to delve into the connection between awakened sleep and higher states of consciousness. Here,
we'll ask you to consider a variety of new practices to implement on your
path to health, happiness, and enlightenment. We will dive further into
Vedic wisdom to help explain how sleep connects us to deeper realms of
our experience, often shedding light on factors that elude modern science. In this chapter, we start with a multisensory consideration of sleep
and the sleep environment.

As you learn about the importance of the senses and sensory input, you'll see why they deserve an entire chapter of their own and an important place in your daily and nightly routines! To help you understand what we mean, let's take a short survey of all the stimuli that you encounter throughout your day, well before it's time to hit the hay.

What are the kinds of auditory information you're taking in (traffic noise, the sound of machinery, podcasts, music, crowds of people, and so on)? What about visual information (phone and TV screens, fluorescent lights and big office buildings, the 24/7 news cycle, etc.)? Do you have time to settle into comforting physical textures—the touch of a loved one as you hold them close, a soft and warming blanket, a soothing bubble bath—or do you move through life without paying much attention to how the protective layer of your skin is interfacing with the world around it? Are you savoring the tastes and smells that come your way, or are you mostly consuming them on autopilot, perhaps not even sitting down to eat a meal or smell the metaphorical and literal roses?

We want you to be as detailed as possible as you consider all that enters your sensory organs during the day. How attuned are you to your senses? What is the general quality of sensory stimulation in your daily environment? What is the impact this ends up having on your body, your thoughts and emotions, and your spirit? It's extremely important to ask yourself these questions as whatever you are welcoming through the gateway of your senses during the day is affecting your sleep at night. And when you don't or can't fully process sensory experiences from the day, you carry them into your sleep. In fact, REM—or our natural dream state—is associated with the emotional processing of our day. And we all know that if we're having dreams that replicate the drama and discord of our waking hours, we don't exactly wake up on the right side of the bed.

Sleep can become challenging when we wake up troubled or go to sleep dreading the stretch of hours ahead of us because our hearts and minds are still attempting to catch up with whatever we experienced. Believe it or not, sleep is meant to be joyful and pleasurable. But when that joy and pleasure are depleted because our senses are sponging up all of life's disturbances, we need to start paying attention to our sensory nourishment, or lack thereof. Is what we're putting in affecting what we're getting out?

In order for us to wind down and reenter the ocean of consciousness that awakened sleep promises, Ayurveda teaches us that we need to pay *a lot* more attention to the quality of our sensory experience prior to bedtime—and by that, we mean all our waking hours. Whatever we haven't completely "digested," including sensory input, will be taken into the night to be processed, which means we won't have the capacity to dive into deeper realms of possibility. That's why this chapter is an exploration of something that should be evident but that doesn't actually occur to many of us: Our sensory experiences from the time we wake until the moment our head hits the pillow influence our sleeping patterns. And science is coming to validate this concept.

The most common issue we see is that people are bombarding their senses to the point of exhaustion. Ironically, a lot of our patients with sleep troubles rely on this technique to get to sleep. You know the drill: binge-watching TV until you fall asleep, scrolling social media and dozing off with your phone still in your hand, blasting your favorite album on your AirPods in a repetitive loop, leaving all the lights on, etc. Such overstimulation of the senses adversely affects the nervous system and can set in motion a train of unfortunate consequences that damage our well-being in the short and long term.

Thankfully, there are sensory inputs that can actually work for you rather than against you. Through an exploration of the power of sound, touch, sight, taste, and smell, both in and out of your sleep environment, you can gain a deeper awareness of how your technology, your daytime and nighttime activities, and your unexamined habits can all affect your sleep. Five-senses therapy (using the senses to facilitate health and restorative sleep, including activities like listening to relaxing sounds, taking a warm bath, dimming the lights, including calming colors in your bedroom, etc.) has greatly supported our patients in breaking out of some of those habits and bringing more peace to the gateway of their sense organs—and knocking on the door to awakened sleep.

THE GATEWAYS TO PERCEPTION

In Sanskrit, *indriya* is the word that most closely corresponds to our senses. This is further described to include sensory organs, or *jnanendriyas*, which include the ears, skin, eyes, tongue, and nose. Another translation for *jnanendriya* is "senses/organs of knowledge," implying that we take in knowledge through these organs. In Vedic wisdom, the sense organs are considered the gateways to the mind as they inform and influence the state of our mind. Moreover, each sense organ is attached to a motor organ that acts out what the mind processes from the senses. These are known as *karmendriyas*, or organs (senses) of action. These are our means of expression and include parts of the body that correlate to speech, grasping, walking, elimination, and procreation, which are ways we interact with the external world. The information that comes into the sensory organs is processed in the mind, which creates our actions in the world, highlighting the importance of paying attention to what's coming in through our senses.

We can make use of this knowledge to help us sleep. Indeed, there are many practices that can help us filter and clarify our perception so that we aren't simply holding on to the negative experiences of our day—something that can have obvious adverse effects on the quality of our slumber.

For example, according to Ayurveda, the foot contains marma points that correspond to different parts of the body. In this model there is a connection between the feet and the eyes, meaning that massaging the feet can similarly calm eyes that have been overstimulated by staring into a screen. Connections between distant body parts are not unheard of in modern medicine. There can be disparate parts of the body that develop from similar embryological tissue cells. For example, in vertebrates (such as humans), a layer of cells called the *ectoderm* subsequently develops into hair, skin, hooves, and nails, as well as the lens of the eye and the lining of the sense organs. So, something that influences one of those tissues could potentially influence another in a distant part of the body. Could it be that ancient wisdom recognized these distant embryological connections? We do know that the nervous system pervades the entire body and can send communication to distant structures all at the same time. This may be one of the mechanisms that result in what Ayurveda has observed for millennia.

The *tanmatras* are another Vedic concept that comes into play when we talk about the senses, as well as the withdrawal of the senses in the process of awakened sleep. The tanmatras refer to subtle elements that preexist the sensory organs themselves; in other words, they're primordial qualities that permeate the universe but can be experienced only through the senses. The tanmatras are the senses of sound, touch, sight, taste, and smell. Each tanmatra corresponds to a specific indriya, or sense organ. You can think of the indriyas as receptors for the tanmatras. As we come into contact with different sensory inputs, those impressions are carried through the sensory organs and into the *manas* (mind), which is what creates our sense of reality—even our ability to differentiate between truth and falsehood—and then informs our actions.

The tanmatras contain the essence of our potential, and they're the basis for the creation of what we'd consider the "gross" elements, or *mahabhutas* (the gross elements of space, air, fire, water, and earth). In fact, the mahabhutas, indriyas, jnanendriyas, karmendriyas, tanmatras, and signs and planets of the zodiac are all interconnected in the Vedic worldview. To put it another way, our individual perceptions are connected to our actions, but they're also connected to larger cosmic cycles and laws of nature.

Through our awareness of the tanmatras and indriyas, we get a sense of exactly how we've trained our senses over the years, and how they can lead to dosha imbalances. In addition, we can train our senses to our benefit as well. There is a process known as neuro-associative conditioning that connects sensory input, especially smell, to a particular emotional state. We have all likely had the experience of a smell bringing back a vivid memory and emotion. For example, smelling a perfume that your grandmother wore may immediately bring you back to the memory of her hugs and a feeling of safety. In this way, when you meditate or listen to calming music, you can apply essential oil or use a pleasant scent in a diffuser to connect that scent to a feeling of calm. Then, in a stressful situation, when you smell the scent, your body and mind respond with the memory of calmness.

This will be a subjective experience for everyone. Some might be more attuned to what they receive through their vision; others might have a keener sense of taste and smell. And when one sense is reduced, another may be heightened; for example, somebody with visual impairment might experience a more acute sense of hearing compared with others.

Sound is considered the subtlest of the tanmatras, and it's the one most closely associated with meditation. *Akasha*, the Sanskrit word for "space," is considered to be the subtlest of the five gross elements and holds the most potential for healing. Sound is the tanmatra that's most receptive to the vibratory impulses that can be found in space. Everything unfolds in space, generating vibrations and sounds that range from deafening to inaudible. The cosmic dust of space is constantly in a process of reorganization, and sound initiates our awareness of that process and actually creates the organization of matter. Deep meditative states can even allow us to "hear" *nada*, which is the Sanskrit term for the eternal background hum of creation itself.

For the dedicated student, there are meditative techniques that help them become capable of seeing, hearing, tasting, smelling, and touching beyond what's in our typical conditioned capacity. More accurately, it isn't that their senses become heightened to the extent that they feel hyperaroused—which implies an anxiety that's caused by stress—it's that their awareness becomes more heightened . . . almost like they're experiencing life as a richer, more textured panorama that helps them notice what many others may not.

The Vedas say that the web of *maya* (illusion) occurs through the external senses, and we are still caught in this web even as we sleep and dream—which can result in something like having a dream in which we're still reenacting all the same actions and behaviors that we did in our waking life. And although sleep is a state of withdrawal from external sense objects, we know that the indriyas and tanmatras persist within us as subtle senses, even in deep sleep.

We can't take away our senses. However, we can pay attention to what we're "feeding" our senses throughout the day, from the time we wake up to the time we go to sleep, much as we pay attention to what we feed our body. This was probably easier for the ancient yogis, who would retreat to their mountain caves to make the world around them disappear. But if you live in Los Angeles, Manhattan, Tokyo, or any other busy metropolis, you can't simply shut out the stimuli of the world. This is why honing our awareness of what we are taking in and how we are responding is so important. Many of our clients lead extremely busy lives. However, it's still possible for them to get back to the cave, so to speak, and enjoy a more mindful lifestyle that permeates the other domains of their existence.

As we try to teach our patients, improper input or overstimulation through our senses and sensory organs can lead to an easily distracted and overwhelmed mind. For example, if we're scrolling social media for several hours a day, we're overfeeding our visual and auditory senses. Whatever we take in through our senses gives rise to our intellect and the nature of our mind and thoughts; when we change what we are taking in through our senses, we literally change our lives.

Ayurvedic practices help prepare us for the effective processing of all the sensory input that comes in, and for restful sleep. But if we're busy processing loads of sensory input we've picked up during the day, or if we're processing unhealthy input, this creates a stress on our entire system. Ayurveda contends that disease is created by improper contact with sensory objects, meaning that we're using our senses in unhealthy ways. We might do this through overuse, underuse, or abuse of our senses, which can create a mental imbalance that leads to physical disease. This also applies to sleep. Sleeping too much or not enough is an example of overuse and underuse, respectively. And if we don't go to sleep at the right time, this is yet another example of abuse.

Overall, we need to figure out the happy medium between over- and understimulation of the senses. Our mind and senses need to be tired enough for us to sleep; otherwise, we'll toss and turn. At the same time, if we're too exhausted, this could lead to depletion and lethargy, which can also interfere with our sleep.

In our modern context, the greater concern tends to be overstimulation of the senses. However, we also have to recognize that we need a certain amount of stimulation, or else we'll lose cognitive sharpness, memory, and other important faculties. Studies have revealed that people with hearing loss have a 60 percent higher risk of dementia. This has also been shown with loss of smell, and most recently, researchers have linked vision impairment with cognitive decline and dementia,[1] which points to the importance of engaging our senses in ways that stimulate neuroplasticity (creating new neural connections in the brain to keep it healthy) without making us feel like we've been run ragged.

Overall, improper use of the senses can lead us to make decisions that affect our physical, mental/emotional, and spiritual health. Ayurveda generally refers to this as *mistaken intellect*, or *pragyaparadh*. This may mean we engage in sensory indulgences that end up harming us. Or perhaps we lack the patience, discipline, and emotional self-regulation to attend to ourselves in healthy ways.

Again, we want to emphasize that our senses are *not* the enemy—in fact, they can be portals to healing. We just need to understand that all information that enters our sense organs must be processed. As the gateways of perception, our sense organs are the threshold between our external and internal worlds. All day long, even when we're not aware, whatever we're taking in is unleashing a cascade of biochemical reactions. The stress that comes from overstimulated senses—and thus, an overactivated sympathetic nervous system—can result in a higher production of epinephrine, norepinephrine, and cortisol. All of these stimulate the mind and body and interfere with sleep.

Understandably, it can be tough to make good decisions when we're activated. And to make matters worse, we take a stressed-out sympathetic nervous system into our sleep, which disrupts our sleep patterns and causes us to wake up even more stressed. In that state, we continue to make choices that generate similarly stressful experiences. Lather, rinse, and repeat.

Science has confirmed that all sensory input connects to and is processed by the nervous system. In fact, we know that all sensory input, in whatever form (sound waves, photons, changes in pressure and temperature, and molecules), is converted into electrical impulses that then travel to the limbic region of the brain (a.k.a. the emotional brain). Sensory input comes into the thalamus and is relayed to corresponding parts of the cerebral cortex for interpretation. But apart from that, as the input first enters the thalamus, it sends signals and communicates with surrounding structures such as the amygdala (which influences our emotional state and reactivity), the hippocampus (which is involved with memory), parts of the cortex (that help us make decisions and move the body), and other structures within the limbic system that can influence our state of arousal (feeling sleepy or awake). The thalamus is situated very close to the hypo-thalamus as well, which may be a pathway whereby sensory information can even influence the release of hormones. So, sensory input can have profound effects on our memory, mood, state of arousal, hormonal control, some aspects of our movement, and our sleep itself!

It can be tough to regulate our senses in ways that allow us to thrive, but we see our patients break out of these vicious cycles every day and learn to make more intentional choices. As an example, Dr. Sheila worked with Jim and Tina, a couple with two young kids, who were struggling in their relationship. Jim was a busy corporate executive who spent the majority of his day managing a large international team and working hard to get important projects off the ground. Tina was a stay-at-home mom who spent the bulk of the day shuttling the kids to school and after-school events and taking care of the household. They lived in a fast-paced suburb with constant street noise; the sound of landscaping equipment first thing in the morning; and loud, talking children all evening.

After homework and dishes were done, the whole family went to bed. The couple retreated to their bedroom, and Jim turned on the TV to get his mind off work. Tina was bothered by the noise of the TV, especially since it was typically tuned to news that made her anxious, so she put on headphones and listened to music to calm herself down from the hectic day. They often fell asleep with the TV on, with Tina waking at night to turn it off. Tina often had trouble getting back to sleep, so she would read until she was tired. The alarm went off too early, and she arose again to the sound of leaf blowers. Jim was already awake and gone for the day. They recognized that they were in an unhealthy pattern but didn't know how to change. They didn't consider that the quality of their sensory experiences was affecting their sleep and their relationship.

The first suggestion was that they tuck their two small children into bed by 8 or 8:30, which would give them time to spend together as a couple. They did the dishes together with no other noise around them, so they found the space to talk to each other about their day. They removed the TV from the bedroom and sometimes watched something light in the living room before bed, but they agreed to be in bed together by 10:30 p.m. They would then go to sleep, not overstimulated by lights and noise, and wake up together feeling more rested and connected.

Jim and Tina followed up a few months later to share that their relationship had greatly improved after incorporating these few suggestions. Although there may be times when a partner is not as willing to make changes as they both were, each person can find their own small ways to decrease the sensory overload that pervades modern life.

A JOURNEY THROUGH THE SENSES

It's a good idea to pay attention to any sensory inputs we're taking in well before bedtime, but perhaps most important is what we are taking in right before bedtime. We don't want to engage with sensory inputs that stimulate our mind and nervous system directly before bedtime, especially because sleep is a period when we want to withdraw our senses from external sensory objects.

For example, Tina mentioned a time when she could hear a neighbor fighting with their spouse, which spurred negative and fearful thoughts about her own marriage—which, in turn, led to disturbing dreams and the feeling of waking up on the wrong side of the bed. Tina recalled going to sleep swirling in a jumble of disturbing thoughts, including her parents' strained relationship and whether or not Jim was having an affair. Tina was going to sleep wrapped in the envelope of unpleasant sensory experiences—all of which had been initiated by hearing her neighbors fight. Needless to say, Tina's primary dosha was Vata, and she was particularly sensitive to overstimulation and worry.

It's not bad to have a sensitivity to sensory input. In fact, it also allows you to use your senses in a therapeutic way. In traditional Vedic cultures, *yantras*, or geometric patterns that are often engraved on copper plates, are complex shapes that are believed to have a calming effect on the mind and body—similar to dream catchers, which in Indigenous traditions are believed to protect people from distressing thoughts and nightmares. When one focuses their attention on these shapes and images, these "assists" can strengthen the mind, which can also lead to greater discipline and the ability to focus our attention and intention in daily life.

The environment we are spending most of our time in can be a wonderful force for sharpening our focus and assisting in a sense of tranquility. When we teach Ayurvedic health concepts, we often use the metaphor of the environment being our extended body. We are in constant exchange with the environment around us; what's happening outside affects us inside. In the context of our sleep, everything in our surroundings—the quality of light, sounds that envelop the room, plants and greenery, etc.—becomes a part of us.

Our physical body doesn't end at the edge of our skin but is very much a part of the elements in our overall environment, even outside the bedroom. For example, the soil that grows our food provides us with the minerals and nutrients that become our body, the water we consume becomes our circulation, and the air outside moves in and out of our lungs. In all ways, we are intimately touched by nature. When we stop to consider this, we can also note that the state of the physical body as we sleep is directly affected by the environment of the neighborhood, the room, the bed, and the people who occupy our bed with us. This is why intentionally creating a restful state right before bed can be so helpful. Even if we have a stressful job or we're experiencing challenges with a family member, we can consciously work to make the bedroom a sanctuary for sleep. And we can ritualize what we do at bedtime, so that we're regulating our nervous system to feel comfortable as we drift off into the ocean of consciousness.

Some of the effects of our bedroom environment are obvious. For example, when the room is hot, we feel hot. When the room is cold, we feel cold. Although many experts feel that a cool room, between 60 and 70 degrees Fahrenheit, leads to better sleep, one study showed that after age 60, sleep improves if the room is between 68 and 77 degrees.[2] This period of life, of course, corresponds to the Vata stage, which requires greater warmth in order to reach the right balance. As your body changes, your environment should naturally follow suit. In addition, people with a primary Vata nature will often be the ones throwing on more soft blankets (or using a heating blanket) when their partner is perfectly comfortable. Ayurveda gives us amazing insight into how to become aware of and adjust to the sensory qualities in our environment so we can stay balanced and create restorative sleep.

Another interesting consideration is your immediate outdoor environment. A recent study of adolescents in Southern California showed that residing in urban areas of greater greenness was associated with improved sleep duration among children of low socioeconomic status.[3] This is likely due to multiple factors, including access to spaces to move, play, and exercise; improved air quality; and connection to nature itself. In a recent review of studies on interventions using green spaces for sleep, findings supported evidence of a positive association between green space exposure and sleep quality and quantity.[4] Considering that more than half of adolescents do not get the recommended eight hours of sleep, paying attention to our environments is important and reinforces the power of facilitating the creation of green spaces in all living environments.

In fact, living in urban environments in general can affect sleep. There are studies that show that living in a noisier neighborhood has been associated with later sleep onset and shorter sleep duration. Some studies even suggest that this chronic, low-grade noise pollution can cause chronic, low-grade inflammation, which can negatively affect physical and mental health.[5]

Air pollution has been associated with both obstructive sleep apnea and sleep-disordered breathing, while a growing body of research shows us that artificial light from the streets at night can increase the risk of not only sleep disorders but diabetes, Alzheimer's disease, and even breast cancer.[6] According to the United Nations, 55 percent of the global population lives in urban areas, and that number is projected to increase to 68 percent by 2050.[7] Paying attention to our environment as a whole will allow the entire planet to sleep better!

As far as your own personal "extended body" goes, it's good to consider the space you currently inhabit. Taking the time to consider your current, as well as ideal, environment, can aid you in thinking more intentionally about how to invite awakened sleep into the sacred sanctuary of your body and your bedroom. Following are suggestions on how to engage with five-senses therapy to create a more supportive sleep environment. Keep in mind that we will all have our own subjective experiences with respect to what we find soothing. For example, you might like the sound of ocean waves, whereas someone else might have stressful associations with the ocean that make it a less-than-ideal soundtrack for sleep. Please customize these suggestions to whatever feels best for you.

ense	Questions to Ask Yourself	Practices for Nourishment	Things to Eliminate
ound	What are the sounds that permeate my day (e.g., bird noise, machinery, traffic sounds, arguments, animated conversations, etc.)? How do these sounds affect me (e.g., create a distracted attention, cause a sense of irritation and anxiety, connect to old memories, etc.)? What are the sounds that give me a sense of peace and balance, whether I encounter them daily or not (e.g., monks chanting, ocean waves, rainfall, a child's laughter, a cat's purr, etc.)?	Chanting. Repeating a silent mantra (the mantra *Om Agasthi Shahina* can evoke deep, restful sleep). Singing devotional songs (e.g., *kirtan*). Listening to soft, soothing music or nature sounds. Listening to binaural beats (which we hear when two tones with barely different frequencies are played in each ear, causing the brain to interpret the difference as a third distinct tone). Rubbing the inside of your ears with a soothing oil.	Music, TV shows, and movies with loud or jarring sounds. Violent or swear words. Noise pollution, such as traffic or neighbors (which might require soundproofing your sanctuary or using soft earplugs). Unnecessary sounds in the environment, such as background music or TV.
ouch	What are the textures and sensations that permeate my day (e.g., a partner's touch, a pet's fur, sharp or inorganic surfaces, chronic pain, silky or velvety clothing, etc.)? How do these textures and sensations affect me (e.g., create a sense of comfort, generate feelings of loneliness or distress, etc.)? What are the textures and sensations that give me a sense of peace and balance, whether I encounter them daily or not (e.g., hugs, a warm bath, squeezing a rubber ball, orgasm, loving self-touch and massage, etc.)?	Sleeping on a good mattress that isn't too firm or too soft. Sleeping with eco-friendly, natural sheets that help regulate body temperature (in cotton or silk, which keep you cool in warm weather and warm in cool weather). Opting for loose-fitting, breathable sleepwear in cotton or silk. Having a pillow that supports your neck. Keeping your bedroom at a comfortable temperature for you. Keeping a weighted blanket on your bed. Taking a warm bath before bed. Self-massage with a nourishing oil before bedtime (check out the breakout box titled "Self-Massage for Relaxation").	Too much exercise in the evening, which can overstimulate and heat the mind and body and interrupt sleep. Synthetic material in sleepwear and bed linens. Toxic material in clothing, such as flame retardants and other chemicals. Skincare products or home cleaning agents with a lot of chemicals and hormone disruptors.

Sense	Questions to Ask Yourself	Practices for Nourishment	Things to Eliminate
Sight	What is the imagery that permeates my day (e.g., screens, social media, highways, an office environment with cubicles and fluorescent lights, beautiful landscapes, etc.)? How do these images affect me (e.g., create a sense of overwhelm or fear, create a sense of inspiration, etc.)? What are the images that give me a sense of peace and balance, whether I encounter them daily or not (e.g., mountains, the ocean, a beautiful sunset or sunrise, art, images of loved ones, etc.)?	Gazing at the horizon at sunset, or the moon and stars at night. Keeping your bedroom dark. Using an eye mask while you sleep. Placing ghee (clarified butter) around the eyes before bed, which has a cooling and moisturizing effect. Doing eye exercises (circling clockwise and counterclockwise slowly, at least seven times). Keeping images of nature in your bedroom. Gazing at images of mandalas or yantras (geometric figures in Eastern religions that represent the universe and create a sense of harmony and order), and also keeping them under your pillow. Placing affirmations and inspirational words around your home.	Music, TV shows, and movies with jarring or overstimulating energy or violence. Light pollution, such as light emanating from plugged-in gadgets, screen time, and/or news right before bed.
Taste	What are the tastes that permeate my day (e.g., fast food, processed foods, alcohol, sweets that people bring to the office, etc.)? How do these tastes affect me (e.g., increase craving, cause a sense of depletion, generate more energy, etc.)? What are the tastes that give me a sense of peace and balance, whether I encounter them daily or not (e.g., green tea, citrus fruits, berries, nuts, dark chocolate, etc.)?	Oil pulling (swishing an edible oil, such as coconut oil, in the mouth before spitting it out). Tongue scraping (removing bacteria, food, and other particles from the surface of the tongue, usually with a copper or stainless steel tool). Eating fresh, plant-based foods. Engaging in eating meditation by savoring your food, chewing thoroughly, and consuming slowly. Drinking a warm glass of milk or golden milk before bedtime (milk substitutes work as well). Drinking water from a copper cup (often used in Ayurveda for its antimicrobial, purifying qualities) before bedtime.	Eating too much or overly heavy food especially in the two hours before sleep. Eating unnatural, processed foods.

nse	Questions to Ask Yourself	Practices for Nourishment	Things to Eliminate
nell	What are the smells that permeate my day (e.g., flowers, meals you cook, "chemical" scents in every-day items, perfume or cologne, trees, garbage, diesel exhaust, etc.)? How do these smells affect me (e.g., generate a sense of repulsion, make me feel more relaxed, etc.)? What are the smells that give me a sense of peace and balance, whether I encounter them daily or not (freshly laundered clothing, lavender and other essential oils, vanilla and other ingredients used in baking, trees, the ocean, etc.)?	Using a neti pot to rinse the nasal cavity and promote respiratory health. Using nasya drops in your nostrils to moisturize and protect the nasal cavity. Keeping a humidifier in your room. Using an aromatherapy blend in a diffuser or on your eye mask or pillow.	Strong or disturbing odors. Pollutants or allergens. Artificial scents (such as those found in many rooms, office spaces, and car fresheners).

Self-Massage for Relaxation

Self-massage in the morning as part of your daily routine is a great way to use your sense of touch to self-regulate and experience a deeper relaxation that you can carry into the rest of your activities. This is known as *abhyanga* in Ayurveda, and it contributes to improved circulation, softens the skin, and serves as a way to hydrate and lubricate the body as the oils are absorbed. It also strengthens your internal organs, tissues, bones, and joints.

Generally, it's a good idea to use a warming oil such as sesame in colder weather and a cooling oil such as coconut in warmer weather, although preference may vary according to your primary dosha. Using a small amount of oil, start at your scalp and massage in a circular motion. Then massage the face, ears, neck, and shoulders. Add more oil as needed, and gradually massage oil into the whole body, down to your feet. You can use long, firm strokes for your limbs while circular strokes are ideal for your joints. Be sure to include your fingers and palms, as well as your toes and the soles of your feet. Let the oil soak in for at least five minutes to penetrate the skin. During this time, you may wish to engage in intentional breathwork, or do some journaling around your intentions for the day. After five minutes, take a warm shower or bath; as your body heats up, the oil will be further absorbed and any excess will wash off. Be careful as you move around the floor and tub as your feet may be slippery; you can also lay down a towel to absorb extra oil.

Doing a daily oil massage nourishes the body and also grounds and stabilizes Vata dosha by balancing its light and dry qualities. A useful time to do a light self-massage is before bed. Using gentle, slow strokes while massaging relaxes the nervous system and releases calming neurotransmitters via the skin, so you can have a more restful and relaxing slumber.

According to Ayurveda, there are also several marma points that we can gently massage in order to experience greater relaxation. Sometimes, in Ayurvedic massages, a special three-metal bowl known as the *kansa* is pressed against the feet after the oil is applied to further tonify and regulate the organs. The kansa bowl contains copper, zinc, and tin, which correspond to each of the three doshas.

TONE YOUR SENSORY AWARENESS

You can do this exercise anytime to increase your sensory awareness. But for the purpose of promoting awakened sleep, it's a good idea to perform this exercise right before bed, ideally as you are lying in bed. During this exercise, you'll be cultivating awareness by bringing attention to your senses. When we bring awareness to our senses, we move our attention away from our thoughts and become more aware of the present moment. We also awaken these channels of information in ways that help us attune to and regulate what we're taking in during the day.

If you're not drowsy after the exercise, you can simply place your awareness on your breath—focusing on the rise and fall of your chest or abdomen, or the sensation of air entering and exiting your nostrils—until you fall asleep.

1. Keep your eyes closed and become aware of your ears. Bring attention to any sounds that you are hearing in this moment. Make a mental note of them all. Simply become aware, without judgment and without labeling or naming any of the sounds. Do this for about ten to fifteen seconds.

2. Now, bring your attention to your skin. Feel any sensations on the skin . . . areas of pressure, or perhaps the temperature of the air. Notice the texture and sensation of your clothing as well as the surface you are sitting or lying on. Perhaps you feel more subtle sensations, such as buzzing or vibration on the surface of your skin. Witness all of this for about ten to fifteen seconds, again without judgment.

3. Bring your awareness to your eyes. Gently open your eyes until they are about halfway open. Keep a soft gaze in front of you. Notice any colors or shapes that you perceive, allowing them to come into focus without forcing anything. Try to simply observe

the forms and textures in front of you. After about ten to fifteen seconds, gently close your eyes.

4. Next, bring your attention to the surface of your tongue. Notice any sensations, tastes, or moisture, paying close attention to the subtleties of this sense. You can gently move your tongue in your mouth to notice moisture, taste, or absence of taste. Do this for about ten to fifteen seconds.

5. Now, bring your awareness to your nose . . . to the air flowing in and out. Notice any subtle smells that you perceive, simply maintaining an open and nonjudgmental awareness for about ten to fifteen seconds.

6. Finally, release all sensations, images, feelings, or thoughts, simply allowing yourself to rest in awareness and following your breath into awakened sleep or into the remainder of your day.

OPEN AND CALM YOUR SENSES WITH BREATHWORK

Apart from focusing on the senses themselves, we can use the breath to calm the mind. In yoga philosophy, which is rooted in Vedic philosophy, *prana* is the Sanskrit word that refers to breath, but it also describes the vital life energy that permeates all of existence, from our bodies to the galaxies, and that carries nature's intelligence to every cell in our body. It's responsible for all bodily and sensory functions and the movement of consciousness itself.

Prana can be increased and expanded in the body through a number of practices, from *pranayama* (the regulation of the breath through specific techniques, a.k.a. breathwork) to yoga *asanas* (postures that allow vital energy to flow throughout the body) to the daily lifestyle choices we make. The free flow of prana keeps us healthy while blockage in the flow of prana causes disease. Through the flow of prana, we detoxify both the body and the mind and keep the sensory channels clear. An important part of the "sensory release" process that we want to engage in before sleep is doing whatever we can to calm the nervous system and process the sensory impressions of the day so we aren't taking them into sleep. Breathwork can aid in this process.

There are many different methods of breathwork, and several of them focus on slowing the breath, which also slows the mind. Slow, rhythmic breathing (five to seven breaths per minute) increases the tone of the parasympathetic nervous system, which is what allows the body to relax and conserve energy—meaning it's crucial for sleep. In fact, if you have difficulty breathing (e.g., you snore, have sleep apnea, or deal with nasal congestion), regular breathwork can improve your breathing control, which can alleviate those conditions. A variety of breathing exercises that tone the muscles in your mouth, throat, tongue, and soft palate can be especially helpful in reducing the symptoms of sleep apnea.

Breathwork is also a time-honored meditation practice that helps us shift into the relaxation response in the body and calm disturbing or distracting thoughts. When we're stressed out, our breathing usually remains shallow, which perpetuates the sympathetic response of fight or flight. When we don't consciously slow the breath, our physiology can remain stimulated and in mild stress mode. However, slow, deep breathing stimulates the vagus nerve—the longest cranial nerve in the body and the main nerve of the parasympathetic nervous system. The vagus nerve affects many of the body's organ systems and functions. In addition, by manipulating the branches of the vagus nerve in the abdomen and chest with our deep breaths, we send signals back to the brain to switch into rest-and-digest mode. When this happens, it can generate a sense of calm and the feeling that we're capable of skillfully responding to our daily stressors.

This is our built-in, natural turn-off switch that we can use any-time to calm ourselves in the moment; we can also do slow, rhythmic breathing daily for ten minutes to gradually retrain the brain and body to remain in a calmer state over time. A great way to stimulate the vagus nerve is deep belly breathing: Breathe in for six counts so that your belly and rib cage expand; then breathe out slowly for eight counts, allowing your ribs to move inward—and compressing your belly button toward your spine.

Breathwork is a great tool for overcoming sensory overload, especially right before bedtime. We can use breathwork to regulate our thoughts; to paraphrase an ancient sutra: "When the breath wanders, the mind wanders." If we're having trouble consciously stemming the flow of thoughts, we can focus on steadying the breath instead of the mind, because when we breathe deeply and intentionally, the mind will automatically be calmed as we drift to sleep.

Breathwork is a powerful way of "turning off the lights" inside, just as we turn off the lights in the room before bed. Dr. Sheila has used this analogy many times with patients who are new to these concepts, and it has helped to reinforce the practice and improve many patients' sleep issues. In our clinical practices, this has been one of the most accessible and effective practices that we teach to patients with sleep issues. They can feel the immediate calming benefits, and they generally find breathwork easy to integrate into an evening or nighttime routine.

An excellent review article published in the journal *Frontiers in Human Neuroscience* highlights and summarizes the physiological and psychological correlates of various types of slow-breathing practices.[8] The researchers discovered something that yogis have known for eons—that these practices lead to feelings of increased comfort, relaxation, pleasantness, vigor, and alertness, as well as reduced symptoms of anxiety, depression, anger, and confusion.

Because prana has both an individual and a cosmic manifestation, this kind of deep, rhythmic breathing is associated not only with the parasympathetic nervous system but also with the rhythms of the moon. The *hatha* in hatha yoga comes from the Sanskrit words *ha* and *tha*, which refer to the sun and moon, respectively. The entire purpose of hatha yoga is to use asana and breathwork to balance the solar and lunar channels of the body so that we build the kind of stability that prepares us for higher states of consciousness. Since activity is associated with the sympathetic nervous system and solar energy, practices for awakened sleep tend to focus more on the lunar channel of the body, associated with a more cooling energy, to help us maintain balance. As we switch off from the outer world, we illuminate an inner candle of awareness to induce rest and higher states of consciousness.

Swara Yoga—the Cosmic Breath

In Sanskrit, the word *swara* translates to "sound" or "breath." It can also refer to the continuous flow of breath through one nostril. It's connected to our individual breath but also to the cosmic breath that characterizes the movement of the sun, moon, and elements. The ancient text known as the *Shiva Swarodaya* describes the art of swara yoga, which emphasizes the power of using one's breath to attune to the cosmic breath and to heal illness. The text specifically describes the study and control of breath, which can help us achieve states of consciousness that liberate us from the hold of the distracted "monkey mind," which often interferes with sleep.

In swara yoga, you pay attention to which of your nostrils you are breathing through at any given time and align your activities accordingly. In fact, we go through natural cycles where one nostril is more open than the other, usually every 2.5 hours, although this can vary. The *Shiva Swarodaya* suggests that breathing through your left nostril is good for activities like meditation and mantra recitation, whereas breathing through the right nostril is ideal for practices that nourish the senses, as well as for rigorous mental and physical activity.

Some of these suggestions align with what science has revealed about the nasal cycle and its connections with each of the hemispheres of the brain. The right nostril connects to the left hemisphere, and the left nostril with the right hemisphere. When air flows through our right nostril, this activates the left hemisphere (associated with logic, speech, quantitative thinking, and details); when it flows through the left nostril, the right hemisphere (associated with communication, emotions, metaphors, symbols, and spatial processing) is activated. It's believed that when we predominantly breathe through the left nostril, our immune system and sleep are improved. We can also practice breathing through both nostrils for balance between the right and left hemispheres, as with the classic yogic alternate-nostril breathing technique.

When we attune to the breath, we are able to control our sensory experience; this is the basis of all healing. If you'd like to change the way you breathe, it's a good idea to switch to sleeping on the side of your body that's more active. For example, if you tend to breathe through your right nostril more often (which is associated with mental and physical activity, since it activates your left hemisphere), try sleeping on your right side; your breath will naturally switch to your left nostril. You can also switch the side you're sleeping on every two hours or so, if you'd like to experience greater balance between both hemispheres of your brain.

THE SUBTLE INFLUENCE OF THE GUNAS

An extremely important Vedic principle that affects how we look at sleep comes in the form of the gunas, which are said to be three fundamental forces that interact to create the whole universe. The gunas are subtler than matter and correlate to various energetic principles. These subtle aspects to our sensory input can have specific effects on the mind and on our sleep. The three gunas, which constitute the basis of all matter, are *tamas* (darkness and inertia), *rajas* (passion and activity), and *sattva* (peace and harmony).

These qualities are embedded in the fabric of creation and live inside everything we experience in the material world. They are specific qualities behind all matter. The initial impulse of creation is thought to have given rise to the three gunas, which also exist in matter at the subatomic level, and in the three doshas—in spin (or the angular momentum of a particle, presided over by Vata), charge (the electrical charge of a particle, connected to Pitta), and mass (the amount of matter in a particle, associated with Kapha). We can also make correlations between the three gunas and the three activities of the autonomic nervous system. Sattva represents the parasympathetic nervous system (rest, digest, healing); rajas represents the sympathetic nervous system (activity and mental processes); and tamas represents the overcompensation of the parasympathetic nervous system, now known as the "freeze" response.

Sattva represents creation—the primal force that sets everything in motion. The associated qualities of sattva include lightness, purity, and peace. And when we cultivate sattva in our lives through healthy living, these qualities are reflected in everything we do. As we deal with the activity of the day, we experience rajas, or the subtle energy of activity. This guna is necessary in order to function in our day-to-day lives as its qualities include movement, passion, and dynamism. But when there's too much activity (which is relative and dependent on the person having the experience), our mind becomes overactive. A rajasic mind can interfere with sleep because we are consumed by our thoughts. When evening comes, we experience the qualities of tamas—inertia, slowing down, and darkness—which are necessary for sleep. However, when we do not have healthy practices to manage our daily stressors, many people may experience too much tamas, which brings about numbness, laziness, and ignorance. But thankfully, through awakened sleep, we can cultivate sattva and bring in its bright, clear, empowering qualities, which help us cultivate tenacity and equanimity in life.

All the gunas are important, and none is better than another as they fulfill different purposes that are necessary for life. Just like the doshas, the gunas influence and regulate both our sleep and waking patterns. As we've described above, one always follows the other, through the day and night—and in our sleep, we cycle between all three states.

While each of us has a dominant dosha, we have more freedom with respect to the guna that dominates our life. We can increase the qualities of any of the gunas through the choices we make, but for awakened sleep, it's ideal to increase sattva. According to Ayurveda, the most sattvic times are the transitions between day and night, sunrise and sunset; interestingly, we experience a surge in cortisol, which is the hormone that signals a sense of awakeness, around 6 a.m. and 6 p.m., the sattvic times. When we start and end the day with awareness, we carry sattva into sleep with us. In fact, it is recommended to spend time outside at sunrise and sunset to increase sattva in our minds. We also dispel depression and sluggishness (which a lot of people tend to feel at these times) by engaging in sattvic activities such as meditation, yoga, and pranayama and eating sattvic foods that are natural and fresh. Causes of mortality are at their peak between 7 and 9 a.m., so attending to ourselves with sattvic activity prior to that can mitigate those factors.

In general, we want to decrease the amount of stimuli we're taking in and avoid too much activity as we move closer to bedtime. If we're filling our senses up with more and more, this encourages the rajasic quality of passion, action, anxiety, stress, and irritation—all of which typically permeate the middle of our day. All activities increase rajas, so it's preferable to slow down, and to minimize or avoid rajasic foods (meat, spices, and alcohol). In contrast, if we're dulling our senses through activities such as oversleeping, overeating, or taking drugs or alcohol, this increases tamas, which can lead to a feeling of indolence and depression. Instead, we can focus on winding-down practices like journaling, meditation, and listening to soothing music.

As we bring about sattvic, awakened sleep, we can simultaneously experience the tamasic heaviness of withdrawing our senses from the waking world, as well as the heavy qualities that are necessary for the body to fall asleep. Remember, sattva refers to light and tamas to darkness. We need a balance and integration of these two gunas to create awakened sleep. Essentially, underneath tamas, we can find a purifying and enlivening layer of awareness throughout our sleep. It's a lot like entering a dark room with a tiny flame that allows us to gently see the patterns of our unconscious mind without identifying with them.

We don't have to follow the unconscious scripts of our life. Instead, we can regulate the conditioned, subconscious patterns we may be operating under, either from early-childhood experiences or previous lifetimes. For example, even if we are predisposed to anxiety because Vata is our dominant dosha, our sattvic awareness can help us transcend our limitations and create new, positive patterns in both body and mind, as well as fresh responses to the world around us.

Again, we can't change the physical tendencies we inherited from our parents, nor can we change our dosha, but we can always change our mental type—from tamasic or rajasic to sattvic. As we engage with practices that bring us back into our natural state, we may encounter some of the same issues as before (e.g., stress, anxiety, worry, chronic busyness, overstimulation), but we'll develop new ways of responding to them.

We'll transcend the veil of maya, so that we begin to express all parts of who we are in their most balanced manifestations.

Candle Meditation

Candle meditation, also known as *trataka* in Sanskrit, is a wonderful way to bring the sattvic quality of sleep into the tamasic sleep state. The flame of the candle offers a point of concentration that calms the mind and cleanses the influences of the day. It's also believed to connect us with our third-eye chakra (in the center of the forehead, between the eyebrows), which the Vedic sciences associate with intuition and clear, unperturbed sight (and insight) and the light of awareness. Research has even suggested that trataka can be effective when it comes to improving the quality of our sleep, as well as for cognitive focus, eye health, and even memory.

Try this brief meditation before falling asleep or first thing in the morning, but avoid doing it if you're too tired. You may wish to try this at the sattvic times of day, around sunrise and sunset. Be mindful and do it for shorter periods of time if you experience any eye strain or discomfort.

1. Ensure that the room you're in is dark, quiet, and free from distractions.
2. Set a timer for one to two minutes. You can do this meditation for a longer duration over time, but work your way up to that gradually.
3. Sit with your lit candle just in front of you, preferably at eye level.
4. Breathe deeply, in and out, three times, settling into a gentle

intention in the form of an affirmation (e.g., "I am calm and re-laxed" or "My body is healthy and vibrant").

5. Now, soften your gaze, gently relaxing your eyes so that you aren't straining.

6. Allow yourself to follow the dancing flame with your eyes. Try not to blink too much.

7. Let any thoughts float through like clouds. Let yourself be mesmerized by this tiny, animated flame that arises from the darkness.

8. If you can, notice the sensations in your third eye.

9. Throughout this exercise, continue to breathe deeply, in and out.

10. When your timer goes off, offer a gentle bow of gratitude to the sattvic flame that lives within you and that you can always ac-cess on your journey to awakened sleep! Don't forget to blow the candle out.

REFLECTIONS

1. Bring awareness to all the sensory inputs you experience through-out a typical day. What are any common themes you notice (e.g., lots of noise, bright fluorescent lighting, sharp corners and edges, etc.)?

2. Which of your senses are underutilized? Which are overutilized?

3. Which specific sensory inputs would you like to eliminate (espe-cially ones that may be contributing to overstimulation)?

4. Identify five actions corresponding to each of the tanmatras (sound, sight, taste, smell, and touch) that you'd like to incor-porate into your own five-senses practice. (You'll revisit these in Part 3.)

List any takeaways from this chapter that you'd like to incorporate into your own sleep-hygiene routine:

_____

_____

_____

_____

_____

CHAPTER 6

)) ● ((

HEAL FROM TRAUMA
AS YOU SLEEP

If tonight my soul may find her peace in
sleep, and sink in good oblivion,
and in the morning wake like a new opened flower
then I have been dipped again in
God, and new created.

—D. H. Lawrence

So far, we've talked a lot about bringing awareness to your sleep habits and some of the things you can do in order to begin the journey of awakened sleep. You've learned to remove factors that are interfering with sleep and to find ways to support your natural ability to sleep in order to stay well. But what do you do when you can't sleep because intense emotions that make it hard to relax and let go are stirring inside, even with some of the practices we've discussed? And what happens if, even when you sleep, you toss and turn and find yourself stuck inside a nightmarish realm where it feels like you're replaying your worst memories and bringing the fears and worries that disturb your peace into fruition?

You're already aware that paying attention to your daily routine and your sensory inputs, as well as cultivating balancing practices throughout your life, can be enough to generate awakened sleep, no matter what your conditions might be. A calm mind enables calm sleep. When the mind is rested, the emotions and experiences of your day can be processed and released, so that you can start anew the next morning. That said, there are certain situations that require a more in-depth look at the emotional states that make it difficult to sleep tight, much less sleep in a way that restores and rejuvenates us.

This chapter explores the ways in which intense emotions and trauma can affect our capacity for awakened sleep. When we can't let go of the hold these experiences have over us, which may be well below our conscious understanding, we can find ourselves suffering from sleep deprivation and bad dreams. We might even begin to feel depressed and anxious. When we aren't properly metabolizing and processing emotions related to painful past experiences, they linger within us and leave their sticky residue, and our ability to quiet the mind is greatly hampered. The body's trauma response, which can be restlessness or pain, can lead to alertness and hyperarousal, which often worsen symptoms of insomnia and other sleep disorders.

Unfortunately, in the wake of difficult or traumatic experiences, it doesn't always feel safe to fall asleep. A majority of people who have experienced significant trauma, such as people in the military, report difficulty with sleep; they have a hard time falling asleep, wake up more often during the night, and experience trouble getting back to sleep.[1] This can prevent the deep sleep states we require in order for our body's restorative functions to take place, which also makes people more likely to develop a chronic disease, chronic pain, and poor mental health. And in the case of children who experience adversity, this can lead to sleep problems,

reduced emotional regulation, and behavioral issues and is even a predictor of future addiction and psychiatric illness.[2]

Here, we want to note that trauma isn't something only people who've
lived through adverse childhood experiences, war, or other painful,
life-altering events are subject to. We've all experienced trauma to some
extent. There are many definitions of trauma, but we define emotional
trauma as something that results from an individual's experience of a
distressing or disturbing life event and overwhelms their ability to cope
with it. It can be acute, chronic, or—in the case of repetitive traumatic
events—complex. Trauma is also highly subjective and dependent on a
person's coping resources and skills at the time of an event.

Throughout life, we all undergo negative experiences that can be
difficult to make sense of and process. Often, when this is the case,
we suppress emotions related to the experience. However, the body has
something called *somatic memory*, which is a memory of past events that
is stored in the body. So, even if we've pushed down difficult memories,
they live on in our physical and emotional landscape. And when we don't
process these memories, they can be destabilizing to our relationships,
our quality of life, and our sleep. In fact, from an Ayurvedic perspective,
the mind is in every cell of our body. The mind isn't only our thoughts
but also represents a larger framework for how we understand and ana-
lyze the world. In some sense, our nervous system, which is constantly
analyzing our environment, would be considered part of the mind. When
we have experienced distressing events, our physical and emotional safety
is threatened and our nervous system goes into a chronic hypervigilant
protection mode and creates a fight-or-flight physiology in the body. This
is one way we can understand how we hold on to trauma in the body, via
a heightened nervous system, and how it plays out in our current life and
in our sleep.

Trauma is an extremely complex topic that could fill several books,
but suffice it to say that it's crucial for all of us to take a deep look

at our own lives and recognize whether we're dealing with unhealed wounds and unprocessed emotions that might be showing up through poor sleep. We know that sleep is often one of the first things to be disrupted in the wake of trauma—in the form of nightmares, insomnia, night terrors, and difficulty falling asleep—because we're spinning in a cyclone of perturbed thoughts and emotions and an overactive nervous system. Remnants of the past may contribute to recurring nightmares, and when our sleep time is spent reliving the past, it makes it more challenging to process our current experiences, meaning emotional stress builds over time.

We're not always attuned to our repressed emotions, especially if they're related to deeply buried experiences. Awakened sleep helps us to digest and metabolize the sensory experiences of our day, but it also helps us to bring that which is buried to the surface; to make the unconscious conscious. It helps us cleanse ourselves of strong emotions that may affect us in our lives and continue to reverberate through the night and the day. The five-senses therapy we offered in Chapter 5 is very useful in the process of releasing stuck emotions when they begin to surface. And the Vedic perspective goes beyond the physical and mental/emotional response to our experiences by grounding us in a spiritual understanding of how we can process trauma and suppressed emotions.

Reentry into the soothing, restorative womb of sleep, a place where we can experience safety and a connection to the spirit that flourishes beyond our most painful experiences, can contribute to our healing. It can also repattern our nervous system so that we might process our emotions in a new way and move through challenges without damaging our health and well-being. Please remember that no matter what you've been through, there is light at the end of the tunnel—and awakened sleep can facilitate your process of coming back to yourself and to your natural state of peace and joy.

VEDIC APPROACHES FOR EMOTIONAL RESTORATION

In Vedic terms, trauma can be seen as blockages, or knots, in the flow of consciousness. When we are stuck in the field of maya, we can't fully access the qualities of consciousness, such as compassion, love, and peace, which allow for more expanded perspectives. In general, the mind is attached to experiences with limited perspectives, full of judgment and fear. We are stuck in habitual patterns that we may believe are keeping us safe and in control, but the lack of "flow" disables the capacity for healing. Unfortunately, if we've experienced trauma, the impact of remaining stuck in the field of maya and old thought patterns can be especially painful.

In the Vedic perspective, our experiences of trauma are very much connected to *karma*, a term that simply means "action." When one considers the possibility of the recycling of experience, we can bring the seeds that were planted through the actions of past lives into our current life. But this doesn't mean that we are helpless in the face of a predetermined fate. Many of the practices you've already learned that are directly related to awakened sleep help us cultivate a stronger sense of our full potential and give us the ability to reclaim our choices for the future as opposed to simply living out the past.

Thankfully, it isn't what has happened to us that determines who we are or who we can become. When we are in a more awakened state, which allows us to pierce the veil of illusions and see things as they are with clarity, life's inevitable ups and downs (as well as the more debilitating challenges) don't wound our deeper sense of self. We are able to move past the illusion that our fate has made us who we are or that it's fixed. Awakened sleep facilitates this process as it connects us to our source of consciousness.

From an Ayurvedic perspective, the body/mind/spirit model is integral to the understanding of trauma. Although the nervous system and trauma are described within the paradigm of Ayurveda in a different way than modern science construes these factors, there are some important overlaps. For example, neuroscience has helped us understand that the vagus nerve plays a fundamental role in trauma recovery because it's a key part of the parasympathetic nervous system, which helps regulate the body's response to stress and trauma. Researchers have postulated that by combining conventional trauma therapies with vagal-nerve stimulation, we can harness the power of neuroplasticity to create new, more adaptive responses to past traumas.[3] In the modern context, this involves the use of vagus nerve stimulators (electrical impulses that stimulate the vagus nerve). In fact, a 2024 study published in the *Journal of the American Medical Association* using transauricular vagus nerve stimulation (electrical impulses applied to specific areas of the outer ear) concluded that weeks of treatment significantly reduced the severity of insomnia—and benefits were sustained for up to twenty weeks.[4]

Remember, the nervous system needs to feel safe in order for us to relax enough to sleep restfully. A calm nervous system leads to a calm mind and calm sleep. However, stress and trauma can train us to interpret almost everything in our environment as unsafe. But it's not enough to just tell the nervous system to calm down. This is where Ayurvedic practices come in handy.

The Sanskrit name for the vagus nerve is the *pranadha nadi*, which can sustain and regulate the flow of prana in the body. Prana is the life force that moves both the mind and body and carries pure intelligence, or consciousness. Prana and the breath act as a bridge between mind and body. The movement of prana is responsible for all bodily functions; when prana is blocked, it creates disease, but when it's able to flow freely, it creates health. Trauma results in a sense of contraction within the nervous system that disables that flow.

The vagus nerve is the bridge between the parasympathetic nervous system and the brain and can result in neuroplastic changes and allow for new cognitive pathways to process trauma. Thankfully, we can increase our vagal tone through simple practices like humming, chanting, sing-ing, and even gargling, all of which utilize the muscles at the back of our throat, which can modulate the vagus nerve. When we stimulate, or tone, our vagus nerve, we calm our nervous system, flip the stress response, and soothe an overactive amygdala. In addition, even if we've undergone highly stressful experiences, intentional practices can help dissipate the impact of trauma on our lives and our sleep.

Polyvagal Theory, developed by Dr. Stephen Porges more than a decade ago, is a model that can track trauma's impact on the nervous system. It explains how the vagus nerve is involved in our emotions, behaviors, and social interactions. By understanding the evolutionary development of the autonomic nervous system and vagal pathways, specific techniques can be utilized to heal trauma more effectively. Many of these techniques involve shifting the nervous system from a feeling of fear to safety by modulating the vagal-nerve pathways, thus supporting homeostatic func-tions in the body.

Many of the practices that increase vagal tone, which we'll discuss a bit later in the chapter, are about rebalancing the nervous system, rewir-ing the brain, and transforming our very mind. Here, let's pause and talk briefly about that powerful concept that we refer to as the "mind." This is not merely a description of our mental state (thoughts and emotions), but also the subtle force that influences our embodied experiences, our behav-ior, and our karma itself. The concept of mind includes our thoughts, feelings, and emotions, along with our intellect, beliefs, memories, and judgments. According to Vedic philosophy, the mind is the inner instru-ment that can also be recognized as our sixth sense, more subtle than the five tanmatras, or bodily senses. It's an instrument that can plant the impressions of the external world inside our consciousness. It's actually believed to be rooted in the heart (where it serves as the ultimate arbiter and witness of our experiences, perceptions, and choices) and influences every cell in the body. When the mind is in its optimal state, it is not limited. It is capable of expansive states of awareness and understanding. This ultimately means that its ability to heal itself is unlimited.

According to the Vedas and Ayurveda, there are three types of minds: *pravar sattva*, which translates to a resilient mind that is capable of bouncing back from adversity; *madhyam sattva*, which describes a medium level of resilience that may need extra support in order to move through challenges; and *avar sattva*, which describes a nonresilient mind that causes us to dwell on our problems. Most people fall somewhere in between these, although both trauma and poor-quality sleep can chip away at our capacity for resilience, which is literally the ability to spring back from a stressful or contracted situation.

When we don't get a good night's sleep, we move from high to low resilience, making our mind more susceptible to distressing stimuli, painful memories, and debilitating emotions. We can build resilience when we are fully able to process our trauma—but when we don't, we end up feeling retraumatized, as we reenact our pain and suffering in the domain of the conditioned mind and emotions. Lack of sleep can alter the trajectory of our mind and make us more susceptible to stress and trauma, but at the same time, stress and trauma can result in poor sleep, causing a vicious cycle to repeat. Similarly, we need to engage with healthy practices during the day in order to access restorative sleep, and we need restorative sleep in order to be healthy.

We know that resilience is tied to post-traumatic growth, which constitutes the positive changes we might experience in the wake of trauma—something that many of our patients have directly encountered. When we balance the mind and expand awareness, trauma has an opportunity to resolve. Practices for awakened sleep are all about empowering us and ensuring that we are able to connect to our inner truth, which transcends our external circumstances. When we reenter the womb of sleep, we develop an innate sense of safety that helps us go deeper within, heal our deepest wounds, and access the peace that is always available to us.

SLEEP AS A REMEDY FOR TRAUMA

There are a variety of medical theories related to how exactly we process unresolved or traumatic memories during sleep. It is believed that REM sleep, during which we dream, facilitates emotional processing. During REM, there are changes in neural connectivity in certain areas of the brain—the prefrontal cortex, amygdala, and hippocampus—that help us with processing and consolidating memories, which may assist us in developing new perspectives on memories and separating emotions from experience.

For example, perhaps you can remember a time during which you felt acute embarrassment. However, if you've effectively processed the memory, you won't feel embarrassed as you think back on it; that is, you are able to separate the actual felt sensation of embarrassment from the event. If proper emotional processing hasn't happened, though, you may reexperience that same embarrassment, in much the same way trauma survivors can feel retraumatized when they have an experience that might feel emotionally similar to the traumatic one they went through in the past—almost as if they are reliving it on a physiological and emotional level. The idea here is that if our REM sleep is disrupted, so is our ability to create a sense of significant emotional distance from the past. We might continue to feel unsafe and *triggered*, which is a term that describes an involuntary (even unconscious) recollection of a past trauma that leads to a physical and emotional response. That trigger might even come from something as innocuous as a song, a scent, or seeing someone who bears a resemblance to a person we associate with the trauma.

Ironically, we know that medication for the treatment of trauma can sometimes disrupt our REM sleep. In the treatment of post-traumatic stress disorder (PTSD), propranolol is used to reduce symptoms of fast heart rate, high blood pressure, heart palpitations, and even anxiety, as it has a calming effect. However, we know that propranolol can block the release of melatonin, which is crucial for inducing and maintaining REM sleep. Other classes of drugs used to treat the depression or anxiety associated with trauma, such as SSRIs, are also known to affect REM sleep.[5]

Please be aware that if you're taking certain medications for the treatment of trauma, that doesn't mean you have to stop. It's important to get all the support you need, but we want to emphasize that awakened sleep comes from caring for all aspects of your well-being: physical, mental/emotional, and spiritual. When we are relying on multiple resources to help us with processing trauma, it becomes easier to get to the underlying causes of our suffering—which also means that we can gradually wean ourselves off the things that may be inadvertently contributing to it as well.

An interesting area of research is in a process known as targeted memory reactivation (TMR) during sleep. This is a noninvasive tool that can manipulate memory consolidation during sleep. While further research is necessary, TMR is currently being studied for several potential uses, including learning and dream content, as well as promoting the loss of certain memories, which may have potential in the treatment of PTSD.[6] Interestingly, TMR uses sensory cues, such as sound and odor, to influence memory during sleep, utilizing the connection of the senses to the brain to influence the mind.

Safe and Sound—an Emotional-Release Process

The following practice is especially helpful when it comes to settling the nervous system, creating an intention for healing, and opening the doorway to awakened sleep. This practice was originally developed by Dr. Deepak Chopra and Dr. David Simon, and we've used it for many years with our clients to help them release stored emotions.

We don't recommend doing this practice at bedtime, which may inadvertently bring up unsettling thoughts, emotions, and memories.

The act of engaging in emotional release is bound to dredge up some of our "stuff," and this is a natural part of the process. However, we can be gentle with ourselves as we engage in emotional release, recognizing that we aren't doing it to feel good or bad but to let stagnant old emotions move through us rather than stay stuck.

If you become aware of strong emotions during the day, we suggest taking some time at the end of the day, well before bedtime, to fully digest and release whatever is present. This can help you process surface-level emotions, which can be released first, before uncovering deep-seated emotions from trauma. There may be further work that needs to be done, or a more intensive emotional-release process that is guided by a trusted professional, but this will be a helpful initiatory step on the journey to healing and emotional freedom.

1. Sit comfortably and close your eyes. Allow your awareness to permeate your body, noting any sensations, thoughts, or emotions that are present right now.
2. Gently let your attention rest in your abdomen and heart. Take a couple of full, deep breaths into your belly and notice any sensations you feel.
3. Next, allow yourself to remember a recent event that was upsetting to you. It could be an argument with your boss, being cut off on the highway, or someone being rude to you in a different way. Don't choose a situation that created a huge upset. Rather, recall some relatively minor upset that happened within the last two weeks, bringing the specific details into your mind.
4. Allow yourself to experience any emotions that arise for you around this incident—anger, frustration, sadness, fear, helplessness, etc.—clearly naming and identifying them.
5. Regardless of the circumstances, regardless of anyone else's behavior, these feelings are happening in you and are therefore

your responsibility. Acknowledge that this responsibility is an opportunity and a great privilege, because it means that you have agency. Make a commitment now to take responsibility for your own emotional reactions.

6. Take a deep breath, and once again bring your awareness into your body. Where do you feel the emotion? Your heart? Your stomach? Your neck? Your lower back? Once you have localized the place in your body where the emotion is lodged, breathe into that area while you witness the sensation. Notice that the emotional charge begins to dissipate by simply bringing your attention to it, with the intention to release it with each breath.

7. Open your eyes and take out a pen and your journal or a piece of paper. Express in writing how you felt about the incident, and any emotions that remain. This will be kept completely private, so be open and honest. Use language that accurately conveys what you are feeling. If memories of similar situations come to mind, write about them as well.

8. Stand up. To discharge the emotions from your body, take a deep breath in, raise your arms above your head, and on the exhalation, drop them while making the sound *ha!* You can also shake your whole body, or move in whatever way feels natural to you.

9. Acknowledge the release of the emotion as you perform the movement. Close your eyes if you feel comfortable doing so, and let yourself engage fully.

10. Now, once again, close your eyes and savor the sensations in your body. Perhaps you feel light, or buzzy, or calm, or clear.

11. Open your eyes and slowly bring your awareness back into the room.

You can use this process whenever you notice yourself reacting to anyone in your life—your partner, your boss, your best friend, or a clerk at the grocery store. Although these people's actions might push your buttons, it is usually true that our reactions are related to an incident from long ago—as well as a belief that became a byproduct of that incident. For example, if a parent or caregiver yelled at you when you wanted to play with them and they were busy doing something else, you might have felt embarrassed or humiliated, which may have led to a belief like "I'm a nuisance or inconvenience. My needs are not important in the face of others' needs." This can play into your current emotional state. In fact, most of our current emotional turbulence comes from some experience or belief that we have internalized from the past.

When we view our emotional reactions as opportunities to heal unresolved issues from our past, we stop blaming others for our feelings. As a result, we feel more empowered and more alive. We become compassionate witnesses to our own emotional and mental processes, and we recognize that we have the power to make choices that shape our lives for the better.

RECLAIM PEACEFUL NIGHTS: TRAUMA-INFORMED SLEEP SUPPORT

Dr. Suhas worked with a fourteen-year-old girl, Stephanie, who came to him with her parents because she had difficulty sleeping and was experiencing acute anxiety. Every little noise would wake her up and send her into a spiral of fearful thoughts. This followed her during the day, as she experienced extreme paranoia and an overall lack of safety. It was only through some deliberate inquiry that he discovered that one of Stephanie's hobbies was listening to a true crime podcast about criminals with sociopathic and psychopathic tendencies—right before bedtime. Unfortunately, her parents didn't know she was doing this and hadn't thought to ask about her habits preceding bedtime. As we've previously discussed, sleep helps us detach the mind from the sense organs, but as long as the senses remain connected to the mind, we create a sort of field around the more intense emotions and thoughts that influence us prior to sleep.

He encouraged Stephanie's parents to take her phone away, place her TV outside her bedroom, and restrict her iPad usage. He also gave Stephanie some Ayurvedic herbs for sleep. Beyond this, he suggested that her mother sleep with her in her bedroom for about two weeks. The family was resistant at first, but they quickly discovered that it was instrumental in creating a sense of safety that could allow Stephanie's nervous system to relax, which was being overstimulated and in a state of fear. For Stephanie, listening to those particular podcasts served to inform her nervous system that she was not safe (sometimes, our nervous systems can't always distinguish actual threats from those that feel real). For Stephanie, using touch and the safety of mom at bedtime, as well as removing the inciting factor, allowed her nervous system to regulate, and she began sleeping better.

In the case of an experienced trauma, using sensory relaxation through somatic practices can facilitate a smoother experience of both sleep and emotional processing. For example, yoga is a powerful practice that reconnects us to our bodies, calms the nervous system, and helps us feel safer—which enables deeper sleep. Although rigorous studies on the topic are few and far between, meditation and yoga have been suggested as powerful methods for treating PTSD.[7] Similarly, the controlled rhythmic breathing associated with yoga postures has been used as a treatment for PTSD among military veterans.[8] Further studies are ongoing, and we suspect these practices will become standard of care in the treatment of trauma. And although this research is important to inform medical treatment standards, we encourage you to explore these practices for yourself and see how you respond. We have seen many patients over the years whose sleep and overall emotional and physical health have improved from meditation, yoga, and other Ayurvedic practices.

In the context of Ayurvedic practices, massage and bodywork are especially effective for calming the nervous system. We have previously mentioned the Ayurvedic treatment shirodhara, which we have observed can be quite powerful in aiding sleep. Studies on shirodhara suggest that its capacity to calm the nervous system can lead to deeper sleep; however, the benefits transcend simply calming the nervous system. From an Ayurvedic perspective, gently pouring oil over the third-eye chakra in the middle of the forehead balances the right and left sides of the body and allows the other energetic centers to calm down. This sense of union and synergy is the entire purpose of shirodhara. In some ways, we could say that the emotional and cognitive sides of the brain and body are harmonized, which creates a sense of calm and balance.

When Dr. Suhas worked in his panchakarma clinic, he had a patient, Jim, who had never received bodywork or massage but had come to him due to the benefits he had seen the treatments have on his wife. Jim had trouble sleeping, so he received a shirodhara treatment that he didn't finish—before it concluded, he ran out of the room without saying anything and went home! Dr. Suhas followed up to see what had happened. Jim explained that he'd had an extremely traumatic childhood. In his teenage years, he got into a physical altercation with his father and left home at the age of sixteen or seventeen, never to see him again. Jim explained that his father had died many years later. He was deeply disturbed during the treatment, as he said that he'd literally felt his father's presence; according to Jim, his father sat next to him and lovingly caressed his hair. Of course, the therapist was doing this in order to let the warm oil collect in Jim's hair, but Jim was convinced that it had been his father. After that, he went home and cried all night—something he had never done in his life. This could have been a powerfully cathartic process for Jim that may have led to a remarkable emotional reckoning. After all, he had buried the trauma of his childhood in a way that had fueled his professional success and desire never to be subordinate to anyone else.

Although he was successful, he was embittered, disconnected from his emotions, and not sleeping well (which he knew could affect his overall health). However, given the chance to continue treatments and delve into these stored emotions, he chose to keep them suppressed as the discomfort of strong emotional experiences lends itself to leaving them buried.

Practices like shirodhara take us into the deepest spaces of our subconscious mind. This isn't always comfortable. If we are dealing with suppressed emotions, facing what we have concealed even from ourselves can bring up memories of fear that activate the nervous system. However, if we embrace this as an opportunity to process whatever we have blocked, we can face the emotions that arise, release them, and allow ourselves the opportunity for awakened sleep and an awakened life. As Patanjali's *Yoga Sutras* state, the antidote to fear is trust and faith. Rather than reliving our trauma, we can strengthen our mind and face it in ways that facilitate reentry into our lives.

Breath of the Ocean

Ujjayi breath is a powerful yogic breath that translates to "breath of victory" and "breath of the ocean." You can do this breath on your own very easily; simply constrict the area at the back of your throat so that your exhale sounds like a whisper, a hiss, or the sound of the ocean itself. This sound serves to relax you and to keep you focused and present, especially as you practice yoga, and to bring yourself back into your body (an anchoring practice that is especially useful for people who experience disassociation from their bodies in the wake of trauma).

Ujjayi breath is a powerful method of somatic release, enabling us to let go of lingering tension and to process difficult emotional experiences. When we use this breath, we access our deeper resilience and strengthen our mind. Ujjayi breath creates a harmonious pattern that's akin to the rhythm of the tides moving in and out of the shore of waking life and reconnecting us to all that is. Our breath begins to synchronize with our body's patterns and movements if we're engaging in yoga, which creates a greater sense of fluidity and emotional flow—letting emotions come and go, breaking at the shoreline, and retreating back to the ocean of consciousness.

Several studies have noted the way in which ujjayi breath activates the vagus nerve and the parasympathetic rest-and-digest system. When we use this breathing technique regularly, we get into the habit of releasing emotional blockages and disruptive thought patterns that might cause us to feel helpless in the face of life's changing circumstances, and the benefits are sustained.

Yoga philosophy also notes that ujjayi breath can clear the *nadis*, the energetic channels in the body through which prana flows. This means that emotional blockages are able to drain away from us with greater ease, which also improves our health, vitality, and capacity for awakened sleep.

Here's a simple, step-by-step practice for engaging ujjayi breath to regulate your nervous system and aid in clearing blocked emotions:

1. Sit or stand in a comfortable position, with your body upright yet relaxed.
2. Close your eyes and center yourself with a few deep breaths. Try this for ten cycles of breath, and feel yourself becoming more present.
3. Breathe deeply through your nose, holding briefly at the top of the inhalation.
4. Exhale very slowly through your nose. As you do this, feel yourself gently constricting the muscles in the back of your throat. As

you breathe out, you'll hear it as a slight whisper or hiss. Breathe
out all the air that's in your lungs before you take another cycle
of breath.

5. At first, try this breath for at least ten cycles, inhaling and ex-
haling for about five seconds each. Gently allow your attention
to rest on the sensations of the breath coming in and going
out, as well as the sound of your exhalation, which should feel
very soothing. You may want to visualize waves breaking at the
shoreline and retreating back into the sea . . . imagining that they
are much like your thoughts and emotions, coming and going
like the ocean's tides.

You can do this practice shortly before bedtime, either in a simple meditation or during some relaxing yoga poses. You can also
practice ujjayi breath for a few cycles anytime you feel agitated or
when your nervous system is frazzled. Over time, you can increase
the duration of your practice, which is especially soothing in the
moments before sleep.

REFLECTIONS

1. How might your quality of sleep be related to difficult emotions or traumatic experiences that you have not fully processed? Consider the things that keep you awake at night, as
well as the sleep challenges you're having (e.g., night terrors,
insomnia, waking up in the middle of the night thinking about
troubling moments from the past, difficult dreams or nightmares, etc.)?

2. What supportive practices from this chapter would you like to commit to, during the day as well as before bedtime, to help you process these experiences?

3. Please remember that if you've experienced acute trauma or stressful experiences you haven't been able to process, it's a good idea to seek extra support in the form of therapy, bodywork, or somatic practices that help you move any stuck energy and soothe your nervous system. Be emotionally honest with yourself here. Do you need that extra support? If so, what steps can you take toward finding it? Who can assist you in this process?

List any takeaways from this chapter that you'd like to incorporate into your own sleep-hygiene routine:

_____

_____

_____

_____

_____

CHAPTER 7

)) ● ((

ENGINEER YOUR
DREAM STATE

Dreams are the guiding words of the soul. Why should
I henceforth not love my dreams and not make their
riddling images into objects of my daily consideration?

—Carl Jung

DREAMS HAVE FASCINATED US SINCE TIME IMMEMORIAL. LIKE SLEEP,
they're part of a wildly mysterious terrain. How in the world do we
have such vivid, multisensory experiences when our body is in shutdown
mode?

In general, *dream* is a word used to describe an experience of images,
sounds, ideas, emotions, or other sensations during both the REM and
NREM states, but there is no neurologically agreed upon definition.
Some scientists believe that dreaming (like sleep) facilitates the processing of memories and emotions, as well as allowing us to digest our daily
trials and tribulations. Another neurobiological theory of dreaming is the
activation-synthesis hypothesis, which suggests that dreams don't mean

anything at all. According to this theory, they're an assemblage of electrical impulses that pull random thoughts, memories, and images from our brain's data bank—for no discernible reason.

On top of all this, the stories we create to make sense of our dreams don't exist during the dream; they come only after the fact. But talk to an evolutionary psychologist, and they might beg to differ and tell you about the threat simulation theory, which posits that dreaming is a defense mechanism that helps enact potential threats in our mind's eye—to prepare us for the possibility that they might happen in real life!

Still . . . this doesn't begin to explain *why* we dream. Our current paradigm of study, which relies on the theory of primal matter and fixed natural laws, cannot be used to study a state of awareness in which the material laws of the waking state don't exist. And given the historic disconnect between body, mind, and spirit in the Western medical paradigm, dreams are often discussed only in a pathological context, especially in light of the many dream disorders that scientists have studied: nightmare disorder (a recurring pattern of frightening dreams that can lead to difficulty with one's executive functions), REM sleep behavior disorder (abrupt and jarring body movements during sleep), rhythmic movement disorder (which can include repeated movements like rocking of the body), and other psychiatric disorders that may lead to abnormal dreams.

Long before the *Diagnostic and Statistical Manual of Mental Disorders* (*DSM-5*) began to classify mental health disorders related to sleep, the Vedic perspective presented a simple correlation between dreaming and our overall well-being.

In this chapter, we offer a brief manual for deciphering the contents of our unconscious mind by examining the symbolic language of dreams. This will include simple interpretations of specific types of dreams, as well as how the information they convey can clue us into our specific dosha imbalances. We'll also give you some tips for "incubating" lucid dreams, improving dream recall, and using your dream state to experience pure consciousness. In fact, the field of dreams may hold knowledge and wisdom that transcends our previous ideas; it can enable us to tap into our deepest desires as well as the greater cosmic reality.

DREAMS IN VEDIC THOUGHT

The words *sleep* and *dream* are generally used synonymously in Vedic literature. In Sanskrit, *svapna* is the word that represents the state of dreaming, but it transcends our nighttime dreams. It's a phase of awareness we can experience awake (e.g., while engaging in rumination, memory, or fantasy) or asleep, when we're not able to take in the world around us through our senses.

Svapna is symbolically connected to the moon and the element of water, as well as the tissue known as rasa (related to the fluids inside the body, and the fluid nature of dreams). According to Vedic wisdom, it is also a state of ignorance of sorts.

The standard way we achieve knowledge, during the waking state, is a process whereby the subjects of our awareness meet our sensory organs, which sends impressions to the mind that are processed by the intellect and become part of our ordinary knowledge. This process is fairly linear as outlined below:

Subject of sensory information ⟶ Sense organs ⟶ Mind ⟶ Intellect ⟶ Knowledge

For example, when you listen to a teacher who is speaking, the sound of their voice comes through your ears and is transmitted to your mind, evaluated by your intellect, and then becomes knowledge.

The means by which this process of knowledge acquisition can occur is absent in sleep, during which our senses are withdrawn from external stimuli, and the conscious mind is inert and disconnected from our sensory organs. Therefore, the standard process of gaining information is absent in dreams. What's actually happening is that residual information from our day and our stored memories come up to be fully processed. Everything we may have heard, touched, seen, tasted, or smelled is still in our sensory channels because it hasn't yet been fully processed. In dreams, the mind is literally creating its own virtual reality that enacts itself for our nighttime entertainment.

As we sleep, we have the opportunity to release some of the unwanted stresses and unprocessed information that we receive throughout our day; we can catalog these experiences to a certain extent through the process of sleeping and dreaming, but we're not necessarily gaining knowledge as the waking functions of the mind are hindered by the veil created by sleep.

At the same time, the ancient sages understood the importance of our dreams, which have the power to offer us information about imbalances and disharmony in our waking lives. The *Svapna Prakashika* is an ancient text that decodes dreams. It delineates seven major categories of dreams:

- the dreams that are based on what we see during our waking life (visually driven)
- the dreams that are based on what we hear during our waking life (auditorily driven)
- the dreams that are based on an amalgamation of our sensory experiences during our waking life (mentally driven)
- the dreams that emerge from our mind's desires and wishes (e.g., the desire for a partner might result in erotic dreams, dreams about partnership, or dreams that fixate on the absence of partnership in one's life)
- the dreams that come from imagination and fantasy (e.g., dreams in which encounters with supernatural beings occur, or in which you're able to act and behave in ways that would not seem plausible in waking reality)

- the dreams that come from deep subconscious/hidden places (e.g., dreams related to past lives, future omens, and influences that might be hidden from our overall awareness)
- the dreams that arise from our primary dosha, as well as any dosha imbalances

Let's look at the final dream category, which can offer a great deal of insight around where we might be able to create balance in our daily overall health. Doshic dreams are revealed through a series of symbolic motifs. Although dreams are certainly subject to cultural differences, the era in which we live, and personal associations, the Swiss psychoanalyst Carl Gustav Jung revolutionized the language of dreams by positing that it is, first and foremost, a symbolic one. That is, he believed that dreams are symbolic communications from the individual and cultural unconscious. Most of our dreams aren't purely literal and don't always represent realistic scenarios. Jung wrote, "Dreams are the direct expressions of unconscious psychic activity." He also noted that "it is in dreams that we first encounter the symbol without knowing it as such."[1]

According to Jung, our dreams are filled with symbolic archetypes—or universal themes that transcend cultural specificity. These might include people or other beings that can be personified (mother, hero, angel, demon), representatives of nature (trees, animals, rocks, the ocean, the sky, other natural landscapes), activities (falling, flying), and major themes (death, war, rebirth). In fact, the *Atharva Veda*, from which Ayurveda derives its foundations, contains references to these same symbolic archetypes and emphasizes an interpretation of dreams based on the time of night as well as the individual's life circumstances and physical health. Thus, the content of dreams can include clues to the state of our balance.

For example, Vata dreams tend to focus on experiences of fear, anxiety, and loss. According to the *Svapna Prakashika*, Vata dominance might result in dreams of flying, moving around in the sky, climbing trees and mountains, wandering across vast swaths of land, riding camels or other animals, seeing dried and crooked rivers and trees, hearing rumbling voices, or being exposed to whirling objects. The tendency toward such dreams is more pronounced when Vata is out of balance. Even if Vata isn't a person's dominant dosha, they might have especially frightening or vivid dreams if this dosha isn't balanced. If you're Vata dominant, you're also most likely to recollect your dreams in greater detail. In general, this is because Vata types are light sleepers who tend to awaken throughout the night, which makes it easier to remember whatever they were just dreaming about. Vata folks may seem to have a lot of dreams, and this is also because the act of remembering our dreams can lead to more dreams.

Pitta dreams typically center on rage, violence, and the element of fire. Pitta dreams are often like action movies—filled with adventure and conflict. The *Svapna Prakashika* notes that prominent Pitta dream symbols include fire, flash lightning, the sun, gold, flowers, meteors, golden mountains, entering fire, embracing flames, etc. Again, if Pitta is imbalanced, you might have more dreams with these motifs, or your dream landscapes might be especially violent and wrathful.

Kapha dreams are more pleasing to the mind and senses. The *Svapna Prakashika* paints an idyllic picture: Kapha-dominant dreams often include clouds, calm lakes, ponds, blooming lotus flowers, swimming in the ocean, silver mountains, etc. However, Kapha people are less likely to remember their dreams (note that all of us dream, even if we hold no conscious memories of doing so). If Kapha is out of balance, you might simply wake up with a sense of having traveled through a variety of situations and landscapes, which could end up making you feel tired and heavy.

From a Vedic perspective, food is another sensory input that can influence our doshas and thus our dreams. For example, hot, spicy foods can exacerbate Pitta and lead to "fiery" dreams. Too many cold, dry foods can throw our Vata out of balance and lead to anxious dreams. And foods that are soft, sticky, and heavy can worsen the lethargic effects of Kapha and make it difficult to wake up from the dream state. An Ayurvedic remedy for more sattvic dreams, which balances all the doshas, is golden milk, a traditional elixir made of a combination of milk, turmeric, and other spices. Drinking a cup of warmed golden milk before sleep can lead to more restful sleep as well as dreams that are sweetened by a sense of purity and calm.

The *Svapna Prakashika* notes that not all dreams are created equal. Dreams that we have when we are in a state of sickness, fever, or disease generally have less value, as they arise from intersecting processes in the body as we move toward healing. In many ways, the text (and Vedic wisdom in general) is meant to help people reflect on what in their waking reality might be leading to the types of nighttime dreams they have.

At the same time, the text makes a distinction between dreams occurring at a sensory/mind level versus those that occur at a soul level. Most of our dreams are based on the senses and mind, but they can also occur on the level of the soul (*atman* in Sanskrit). The soul, or awareness, is capable of leaving the boundaries of the physical body behind and visiting different locations. Possibly, you've had the experience of a dream that made you certain you were encountering a past life. These dreams can give us glimpses into a more expanded reality than our waking state allows. Many of us have dreams that leave a profound impact on us. Perhaps this is an instance of our soul taking us into aspects of universal consciousness that, once again, can't be explained by science. At the same time, we can still derive value from even our most mundane dreams, especially if recurring. If one of the functions of dreaming is to give us insight into our waking state, we can do a great deal of fruitful work in the dream space.

However, there are a number of influences that might agitate our dreams and foment a sense of fear and anxiety. For example, some pharmaceuticals that are meant to help us sleep, such as zolpidem (Ambien), can induce especially vivid and disturbing dreams. There are also other causes of disturbing dreams, or nightmares. These dreams typically occur during REM sleep. We usually wake up from them, sometimes in a fight-or-flight physiology, and remember the dream. Severe emotional stressors, including trauma and PTSD, can result in nightmares as we have discussed. In addition, alcohol can disrupt REM sleep and lead to vivid and disturbing dreams.

Sleep terrors, a common sleep disorder, typically occur during Stage 1 NREM sleep, a lighter sleep stage and a transitional state between sleep and wakefulness. They usually take place in the first half of the night, roughly two to three hours after falling asleep. People display signs of intense fear: screaming, crying, thrashing, and sobbing that can last for several minutes. As opposed to nightmares, it is very difficult to wake someone in the midst of a sleep terror, and they typically don't remember the episode afterward. Sleep terrors tend to be most common in children between the ages of three and seven, and they are typically outgrown. In adults, although the cause may be unknown, they can be associated with emotional stress, sleep deprivation, fever, or alcohol.

Another fascinating potential for targeted memory reactivation (TMR) is its role in influencing the content of nightmares. In a recent study using TMR techniques, subjects were told to consciously change the narrative around a recurring nightmare at the same time they were exposed to a sound. The sound was then introduced during subsequent REM sleep periods. Over two weeks, the experimental group reported less frequent nightmares and more positive dream emotions than the control group, and the decrease of nightmares was sustained after three months. This demonstrates another fascinating use of sensory neuro-associative conditioning—something Ayurveda has emphasized for thousands of years, albeit in different terms—to influence sleep and dreams.[2]

Plant Sattvic Seeds Inside Your Dreams

One of the topics we often discuss with our patients who are on a quest for awakened sleep is that we can use the period right before bed to plant seeds of intention that bloom inside both our dreams and our sleeping state. This can become a beautifully proactive way of influencing our dreams with a more sattvic quality. We can literally create meaningful intentions for ourselves before going to sleep.

Whatever experiences and stimuli get stuck in our psyche during the day, we typically end up enacting in our dreams—albeit in a wild, nonlinear way. But what if we were to transform the sensory experiences that get planted in our dreams through a simple process of visualization? Even though our senses are withdrawn from sensory objects as we sleep and dream, the residue of whatever we were thinking or feeling during the day makes its way into our nighttime experiences.

We'll talk more about the power of meditation in Chapter 8, but one practice you can easily implement is engaging in five to ten minutes of visualization prior to falling asleep. What would you like to feel and experience? Maybe you want the experience of feeling confident and enthusiastic while giving your big presentation at work the next day. You can simply visualize yourself as if you're watching a movie on a screen, delivering your presentation with clarity and confidence, and basking in the positive attention of your colleagues and mentors. Be sure to use all your inner senses—sight, sound, smell, taste, touch— to let this vision come alive and touch all parts of your confidence. See this future desired outcome as if it has already come to pass. You can also drop a simple affirmation into this practice. In this scenario, something like "I am clear, strong, and confident" would suffice.

After doing this, simply set an intention to remember your dreams. Most of us gather only snippets from everything we dreamed over the course of a night, which is totally fine. When you wake up in the morning, focus on how you felt, as well as details that pop out in your recollection.

First thing in the morning, write down your dreams and notice if they align with the intentions you set—if they do, you're proving the point that, as the old saying tells us, "Where attention goes, energy flows." If they don't, use whatever information arises for your benefit. For example, perhaps you set the intention to dream about feeling confident during your presentation and then receiving warm accolades and opportunities connected to how successful you were—but instead, you dreamed about being in shark-infested waters. Perhaps your dream relates to a different preoccupation in your life, or maybe it symbolically points to fears you have about "swimming with the sharks" in your work environment. What in your waking life might be connected to disturbing dreams, or dreams that may point to something that hasn't been emotionally processed yet?

Dr. Suhas once worked with a family with a teenage son, Miguel, who was an excellent student and star soccer player. He was in a competitive league but unfortunately broke a bone just a few weeks before a big tournament, which required him to get a cast on his leg. He was extremely sad about the possibility that his leg would still be in a cast by the time the tournament came around as it was his dream to make it to the finals. Dr. Suhas prescribed some Ayurvedic herbs for Miguel—in addition to his doctor's and coach's orders to eat more animal proteins and to take fish oil and bone broth.

Miguel began having extremely vivid dreams at night that seemed to be clearly connected to his desire to participate in the tournament. He had one recurring dream in which he convinced his coach to let him play even though he had a visible limp; his coach eventually agreed, and Miguel was back in the game. The dream always ended in the same way: Miguel scored the winning goal, and his team won the tournament. As he shared this highly detailed dream with Dr. Suhas, it was clear that his waking-life desires were entering his dreaming life in a rather persistent way.

Miguel was adamant—he wanted his cast to be taken off after three and a half weeks, although his doctor had recommended keeping it on for six. Eventually, they all reluctantly agreed to letting him remove the cast on the condition that he'd put it back on if it was clear that his injury hadn't fully healed. Miguel applied healing oils from Dr. Suhas's clinic, and in three days, he was ready to play in the tournament. Remarkably, in uncanny alignment with the details in his dream, he scored the winning goal that put his team over the top—and landed him a prestigious scholarship to play soccer.

Miguel's story is a remarkable example of the ways in which our strongest desires can take root in the subconscious to create dreams that reinforce what we want the most—and even serve as prophetic indications of what is to come. It was almost as if Miguel's dream shifted his physiology so that his body, mind, and spirit were in powerful alignment—powerful enough to overcome his injury.

Of course, not everyone's intentions line up with their actual dreams. We've worked with patients who are wary of setting intentions for fear of recalling dreams that don't completely align with those intentions. For example, if they had a bad dream in which they or a loved one had an accident, they might jump to conclusions and believe they had some kind of premonition that not only will their intention not come to fruition but also something abysmal might occur in the future.

Ironically, while dream recall can be a wonderful method of self-reflection and self-regulation when approached with the right spirit, this is the case only when we're not overly attached. While dreams can be a powerful source of information, it's a good idea never to take them too literally or to place the burden of too much meaning on them. Be gentle and playful with this process. If you have a "good" dream, that's great! Let it contribute to more insight in your day. If you have a "bad" dream, be proactive and tell yourself, "This is good information." Don't allow it to color your mood or cast a shadow over the day ahead as you don't want to unconsciously create some semblance of your dream experience in your waking reality! Don't fixate or obsess on the meaning of your dream. Treat it as a thought that enters meditation by letting it come and letting it go.

LUCID DREAMS: BREAK REALITY IN YOUR SLEEP

One of the most fascinating aspects of dreaming is the phenomenon of lucid dreaming, which is a state of wakeful awareness that we experience in the midst of a dream. We become aware that we are dreaming while we are in the dream. The body is physiologically asleep, yet our awareness, mind, and often memory are intact. Lucid dreaming is one of four substates of dreaming. In fact, it's thought of as the highest or most expansive dream state. This isn't a permanent state, though; we typically go in and out of lucidity in the midst of a dream, and we typically lose that state of awareness upon waking, although the residue of our experience can remain and influence us throughout the day.

What happens inside a lucid dream? Everyone's experience is different, but typically, within our lucid dream environment, our senses are heightened, and everything feels more realistic; simultaneously, we realize that we are the ones shaping, and in turn, being shaped by this version of reality. We can consciously interact in the dream, much as we do in the waking state, but without the same physical limits. Dream-initiated lucid dreaming begins as a pretty normal dream until the dreamer becomes aware of things in their environment that are anomalous. This is when they realize they're dreaming. Wake-initiated lucid dreaming occurs when you move straight from your waking state and into a dream state, without a change in your consciousness or sense of self. Basically, you're entering a dream directly from the waking state with full knowledge that this is what you are doing.

Approximately 50 percent of all people have had at least one lucid dream, although most lucid dreams are quite brief and typically result in waking up. Studies suggest that about 20 percent of lucid dreamers have them on a regular basis, around once a month. Some dreamers have regular lucid dreams, sometimes even every night.

It was only in the 1970s and 1980s that sleep scientists confirmed that lucid dreaming was a real phenomenon, even though it has been discussed in various religious and spiritual traditions for centuries. Participants in a study on lucid dreaming were told to move their eyes in a specific pattern to indicate that they were having a lucid dream; when participants did this while they were sleeping, researchers were able to confirm that lucid dreaming wasn't just an anecdotal phenomenon but something that people are actually capable of.

The majority of our dreams occur in a state of ignorance as we don't know that we're dreaming until we awaken from the dream and recall it. However, in a lucid dream, we can experience a range of possibilities. Some lucid dreamers are able to control the events and people within their dreams, either by affirming aloud that they are indeed dreaming or by mentally directing whatever occurs. Often, lucid dreams are connected to phenomena that may not seem possible in "real" (waking) life, such as flying or teleportation to a different environment, although there are many reports of yogis and enlightened masters engaging in deep meditative practice and achieving *siddhis* (Sanskrit for "fulfillment" or "accomplishment") that grant them seemingly supernatural powers . . . the kind you might have access to in a lucid dream! However, for the majority of us, we achieve these powers only while in our dreams.

Lucid dreams can happen during REM and NREM sleep, but they're most common during REM, when there's a significant amount of brain activity. Some sleep scientists also believe that lucid dreaming can take place in hypnagogic (the moments as we are just falling asleep) or hypno-pompic (the moments when we are just waking up) states, when we aren't entirely awake, but we're not entirely asleep, either.

Lucid dreams may also be more common in people with a larger prefrontal cortex, which is the part of the brain that enables us to rec-ollect and make sense of our memories and to engage in complex decision-making. Such people are believed to be more capable of deep self-inquiry and neuroplasticity. Studies have shown that meditation can increase activity and connections in the prefrontal cortex.[3] As we medi-tate more regularly, it is a natural outcome to become more aware in the dream state, expanding our definition of reality to more than just the waking state. Meditation, assisted by lucid dreaming, might be especially powerful in helping us work through the sticky web of maya and recog-nize when we're caught in illusion. Other research demonstrates that if we are generally open, curious, capable of emotional self-regulation, and creative, we're more likely to have lucid dreams.

Lucid dreams can be beneficial in that they can help us rehearse sit-uations in our waking reality where we might not feel we have much control. Many lucid dreamers report feeling less anxiety and depression, especially because they are empowered to do and say things that they might feel inhibited around in their waking reality. As we'll share in the next breakout box, lucid dreams are extremely vivid and can also result in improved problem-solving and the capacity to tackle problems in a direct way within the context of a dream. They can also garner powerful epiphanies from the characters, landscapes, and situations within our dreams; because boundaries are quite porous in dreams, it becomes easier to seek answers to the questions that might linger with us throughout our day. At the same time, lucid dreams can also pose their own unique set of challenges, especially among people who are experiencing mental health struggles, and especially those who might not be able to distinguish between our shared waking reality and their own individual experiences of reality.

Our heart-expanding night meditation technique in Chapter 8 and our more extensive technique for awakened sleep that you'll find in Chapter 10 are two powerful methods that can help initiate lucid dreaming, as many of our patients have discovered. These techniques can also help readers to transform debilitating dreams and nightmares so they're able to dissipate the effects of the dream state as they reenter the waking state, thereby bringing lucid awareness into every moment of the day.

As you develop restful, awakened sleep, it's likely that you'll have more experiences of lucidity. However, it isn't necessary to force it either. After her mother passed, Dr. Sheila set the intention that she would come to her in a dream, as both her brother and sister had experienced. It took some time, but a few years later, Dr. Sheila had a vivid experience of lucid dreaming in which her mother was present and lovingly caressing her face. As her mother touched her face, she suddenly had the awareness that she was awake in the dream. Just like in a waking state, she had the intention to hug her, and when she leaned in to embrace her mother, she had the direct sensory experience as if she were awake. After a few moments, she slowly awoke out of the dream with the memory of her mom still lingering with her. This experience was distinctly different from simply waking up and remembering a dream. Dr. Sheila notes that she was meditating more frequently during that time, which can open us up to the possibility of expanded awareness—even when we're under the spell of the dream state.

Beyond the Veil of Sleep—Famous Dreamers

The mystical elements of sleep are evident in many stories about major scientific discoveries and creative breakthroughs that occurred as people slept. The subconscious mind has the capacity to work on problems that the conscious mind may mull over exhaustively during the day. Because the subconscious mind is connected to universal consciousness, it opens up a field of pure potentiality that helps us tap into all possibilities and transcend what we have previously known to be true. We can delve into this limitless space of consciousness to find solutions and gain a glimpse into truths that our limited mind and senses may find difficult to grasp within our waking reality.

There are so many examples across time and cultures of people who downloaded powerful information as they slept—whether in a dream or a miraculous recall of something that popped into their awareness in a deep state of slumber. Here are some examples:

- Dmitri Mendeleev, who organized the chemical elements into a systematic and logical periodic table of elements after waking up from a deep sleep
- Alfred Russel Wallace, who developed an early theory of evolution by natural selection after a dream he had in the wake of a series of hallucinations while he was ill
- August Kekule von Stradonitz, who saw the structure of the benzene molecule after dozing off in his chair and receiving a powerful dream about dancing atoms that arranged themselves into the shape of an Ouroboros, or a snake eating its own tail
- Srinivasa Ramanujan, the brilliant Indian mathematician who reported that the Hindu goddess Namagiri appeared in his dreams

to specifically reveal to him a series of complex mathematical proofs

- James Watson, who dreamed of two intertwined serpents with heads on opposite ends, which led him to consider that the double helix was the very shape and structure of our DNA
- Paul McCartney, who woke up with an infectious tune in his head, which would become the melody of one of the Beatles' most beloved songs, "Yesterday"

There are plenty of other examples. Author Mary Wollstonecraft Shelley, poet Samuel Taylor Coleridge, philosopher René Descartes, physicist Niels Bohr, and inventor Thomas Edison all reported receiving powerful messages as they slept. Their stories challenge the notion that our greatest discoveries emerge from our own intellect. Instead, as we enter into the depths of sleep, we recognize that we have the capacity to push open the doors to an altogether different realm—one where the answers to all the questions that we have ever sought exist and are waiting for us to find them.

ANSWERS IN UNEXPECTED PLACES

Perhaps you, too, have had an experience of waking up in the aftermath of a powerful revelation or the answer to a problem you've been grappling with for some time. Sometimes, as we've encountered, people don't always have access to the power of perfect recollection when it comes to pulling those discoveries into the waking realm.

Dr. Sheila once worked with Nina, a forty-six-year-old data analyst who came in for a new patient visit. She often had the experience of falling asleep easily but waking up between 2 and 3 a.m. with an entire program in her head. She immediately sprang out of bed to write it down, but she found it difficult to get back to sleep. It was amazing that Nina was accessing the universal field of creativity while she was asleep, but her enthusiasm in getting up to write down her revelations was creating disturbances in her daily and nightly rhythms. Nina was concerned that if she didn't wake up to write down what had been revealed to her, she would forget it altogether. Dr. Sheila asked her to try briefly scribbling just a few highlights that would help her to recall the rest of the program the following day, yet allow her to fall back asleep.

Once people trust that the received information won't vanish into thin air, they can simply go back to sleep without waking up to write anything down. However, in our current world, our minds are very active, so during the day, the busyness of the mind gets in the way of recalling our dreams and any revelations that may have come to us during sleep. As Dr. Sheila shared with Nina, this is why it is important to maintain a daily meditation practice to release the mundane cares and concerns of the mind. When we do this, we find we can connect to the creative thoughts that emerged when the mind was quiet and we were sleeping. We can also create space for the thoughts to reemerge.

In truth, nothing is forgotten. The subconscious uses a completely different cataloging system, and if what we stumbled upon in our sleep state is truly important, it will reemerge (which is one of the reasons so many people tend to have recurrent dreams—because the subconscious is making it a point to tell us to pay close attention!). Although we tend to use the intellect and the cognitive mind to piece together the vague remnants of information that may have floated to us in the field of pure potentiality, this is not necessary. The field of pure potentiality, which we access in awakened sleep, is a space of infinite creative energy, and it doesn't just fade away. All we need to do is give ourselves more opportunities for unrushed, easeful awakened sleep, which will increase our opportunity to drift back into the ocean of consciousness and receive any messages that may be waiting for us.

VITALIZE YOUR DREAMS

Everyone is unique and likely to find their own route into lucidity, awareness, and sattvic sleep, whether dreaming is a part of that or not. Thankfully, there are a number of ways to vitalize your dreaming. This goes well beyond learning to lucid dream, which isn't necessarily something everyone can do or needs to achieve in their sleep state.

Ayurvedic herbs like brahmi, tulsi, and ashwagandha are great for better sleep, and there's anecdotal evidence that they improve our capacity for lucid dreaming and dream recollection. Dr. Suhas has also made adaptogenic combinations of herbs for his patients that are beneficial for all the doshas. Supplements like magnesium and valerian can be effective as they both induce a state of relaxation and promote lucid, vivid dreams. Of course, our recommendation is that you seek guidance when introducing supplements into your life as it's best to cultivate sattvic habits in concert with taking these herbs.

The best thing we can do for our dream and sleep state is to maintain a nervous system that is clear, refined, and balanced, as we see with meditation. When your nervous system is calm and clear, and when you aren't under any chemical influence, you're more likely to recall your dreams and to have more sattvic ones. And if disturbing or violent dreams come into play, the practices of awakened sleep can help you more easily metabolize and process those experiences from a vantage point of interested curiosity rather than fear. We can do this through the practices in this book, particularly five-senses therapy and intentional daytime activities (e.g., getting enough sunlight, eating a balanced diet for one's dosha, getting enough exercise, etc.). Many of these sattvic practices can also be used to transform chaotic dreams and debilitating nightmares and to help you cultivate a peaceful inner and outer environment, free of distractions and unnecessary stimuli.

Several years ago, Danielle, a patient in her early thirties, came to Dr. Sheila as a new patient. She had complained of abdominal pain for several years and had seen several specialists. She was ultimately diagnosed with irritable bowel syndrome and saw a nutritionist who recommended a specific diet, but nothing helped with her symptoms. She had chronic constipation that, despite probiotics and periodic laxatives, would not improve. In addition, she had developed significant low-back pain, which she had not had in the past. She had experienced depression in college and was now having symptoms of anxiety as well. Dr. Sheila recommended that she start to meditate and do yoga, both of which have been shown to improve anxiety and would also help with her bowel irregularity and back pain. Danielle incorporated both into her evening routine, replacing her habit of watching TV before bed. She was also instructed to eat warm, cooked foods and warm liquids as many of her symptoms were due to a Vata imbalance. She committed to these practices, and two months later, she informed Dr. Sheila that she was having more regular bowel movements and that her back pain had improved. She also shared that during this time she'd started having vivid dreams every night. The dreams would awaken her in the middle of the night, her heart racing. Although the dreams had become less vivid in the previous week, she continued to experience different versions of the same theme. She would dream that she was running, almost as though for her life. At times, she felt as if someone was chasing her, but other times it felt as if she were desperately running toward something, such as a person or a train she was trying to catch. However, she never arrived at her destination. If she caught up with the person, she'd very quickly lose them. And she always missed the train, although in more dramatic renditions of her dream, she'd barely miss being hit by the train.

For a while, she felt as if many of her symptoms were getting worse. She had developed chest pain that was even more pronounced when she was stressed. On rare occasions, she would take a mild sedative to calm the sensation that a panic attack was coming on. Dr. Sheila suggested that she work through these strong emotions by incorporating regular breathing practices and journaling into her life, as well as seeking counseling. Yoga and meditation seemingly had the effect of bringing these subconscious memories into her awareness for the purpose of beginning to heal them. She also began taking brahmi, a powerful Ayurvedic herb that supports awakened sleep, in a ghee form. Over time, this journaling practice shed light on the fact that the dreams were related to repressed emotions she'd been carrying since childhood. She began to recall memories of abuse as a child, memories that had been repressed. As a child, she felt neither supported nor loved by her parents. The sense of constantly running to catch up to someone, but being unable to get to them, had been with her for a very long time.

During the time Danielle came to Dr. Sheila, she'd decided to cut off ties to her family but had no other support system. She began to intentionally connect to a community of like-minded people. She also began seeing energy healers and explored a new realm of healing modalities. Slowly but steadily, she processed and released the suppressed emotions; as she worked to bring greater balance and perspective to her life, the dreams subsided. When she was ready, she even reconnected with her family and now has a relationship with them. Her mood, pain, and physical issues significantly improved, and she began moving forward in her life in ways she hadn't previously known were possible.

Danielle's story is an example of how we can start to realize that the nature of existence is dreamlike—less stable and fixed than we previously thought. By expanding our awareness, we can slowly rewrite the stories that hold us back. As the strong emotions subside, we start to observe our waking and dreaming states with less judgment and more compassion, what sages refer to as "becoming the witness." As a witness rather than a victim, we can be more present to creative solutions and at peace with what is.

In the Vedic framework, waking, sleeping, and dreaming are three states of consciousness that can enmesh us in a limited virtual reality of our own making—or set us free into greater presence, awareness, and health. Sleep and dreams are especially fertile places in which to wake up from the great dream of maya that keeps us frozen in limited paradigms and beliefs, as we are able to access higher levels of awareness. When we realize that the experiences we have while sleeping and dreaming are just as real as those in our waking state, we begin to understand ourselves as more than the physical body, or even the limited mind.

In the Vedic perspective, material reality itself is the illusion. The material world is believed to have been dreamed into existence by universal consciousness (known as *brahman* in Sanskrit). It appears real to us, but it's only one version of reality, restricted by the range of experience that our sensory organs can have. Dreams are the layer of reality generated inside the illusory layer of the material world, so they're ultimately illusory as well, yet not so bound by our sensory capabilities.

Another powerful aspect of vitalizing our dream state is that we start to recognize that we are truly not so separate from one another. We are all consciousness, dreaming a collective dream. As such, we also have a collective nervous system that is responsible for our perceptions when we're awake and when we're asleep. This prompts the question: What is the collective reality that we are all dreaming into existence? Today, it is clearly one of division and strife. Of course, a waking reality that is saturated with fear and separation naturally lends itself to show up in the dream state for us all. This means if any one of us is suffering, none of us can truly be free, as wise people have told us.

How do we generate a new collective dream? As this chapter has shared, it's imperative to start with ourselves; by planting seeds in the collective consciousness that change our waking and dream realities, we essentially contribute to the rewiring of our collective nervous system. This is one way awakened sleep can radically transform our inner and outer landscapes.

REFLECTIONS

1. What is your general relationship to dreams? Do you tend to have Vata, Pitta, or Kapha dreams? Do you typically recall your dreams in great detail, or do you forget them? Have you ever had a remarkable epiphany in the context of a dream?

2. Try the exercise of planting seeds of intention inside your dreams for a full week. What are your general observations? Did this process help you remember your dreams more easily?

3. Have you ever had a lucid dream? If so, recall a particularly vivid lucid dream. What did it reveal to you about the nature of reality?

4. Have you ever had a memorable sattvic dream in which you felt a sense of tranquility and balance even when life was challenging? Take some time to write it down and let yourself vividly recall the feeling of that experience.

5. Finally, take some time to write about a recent dream you had. Don't consult with any kind of dream interpretation manual or dictionary. Rather, use your own intuition and insight to decipher any helpful messages from the dream that can allow you to process unresolved memories and emotions.

List any takeaways from this chapter that you'd like to incorporate into your own sleep-hygiene routine:

_____

_____

_____

_____

_____

CHAPTER 8

)) ● ((

THE SPELL OF SLUMBER—
WAKE UP TO SLEEP'S
MYSTICAL GIFTS

The source of all creation is pure consciousness . . .
pure potentiality seeking expression from the
unmanifest to the manifest. And when we realize
that our true Self is one of pure potentiality, we align
with the power that manifests everything in nature.

—Dr. Deepak Chopra

THERE'S A BEAUTIFUL STORY ABOUT THE HINDU GODDESS NAMED Yoga Nidra (which translates to "yogic sleep" or "effortless relaxation"), who appears in an ancient text known as the *Devi Mahatmya*, a celebration of the great mother goddess who makes everything possible. Sometimes known as Yoga Maya, she is often depicted as a beautiful woman reclining on a couch in a state of repose. In the story related in the *Devi Mahatmya*, the god of creation, Brahma, sits in the lotus within the navel of the god Vishnu, the god of preservation, who is tasked with sending avatars of himself to Earth to provide salvation for humanity. Although Vishnu's sleep is the sleep of pure consciousness, it is aided by the presence of Yoga Nidra to create a state of *sushupti*, a term that describes dreamless, meditative sleep. Brahma implores Vishnu to wake up, for he is the protector of all of creation and needs to save the world from encroaching demons. However, Vishnu remains asleep. And so, Brahma has an idea. He offers what is known as the "Ratri Suktam"—a song of devotion offered to Yoga Nidra with so much praise and devotion that it coaxes her to leave her dwelling place within Vishnu so that he can wake up to defend all of creation. (We include a reinterpretation of the hymn at the end of this book.)

At first, Yoga Nidra says to the god of creation, "You're the creator of the universe, O Brahma. What do you need me for?" He explains, "I need your help in waking Vishnu. Otherwise, he won't be able to care for his creation, which needs him." The goddess of sleep is so moved by Brahma's invocation that she agrees to leave Vishnu so he can stir awake. In the story, when Vishnu awakens, he fights a battle with two demons who have been threatening the manifest world with their treachery. Vishnu ultimately defeats them and praises Yoga Nidra.

It is believed that when we court Yoga Nidra, consciousness comes into perfect balance. We are able to maintain the meditative aspects of deep sleep in a waking state, meaning that we remain serene and at ease as we use our one-pointed attention to slay the demons of the ego and to reconnect with all the vibrations of the universe—and to universal consciousness itself. Yoga Nidra blesses us with her auspicious vision so that we can remain awake and aware even in our deep sleep. She's a maternal archetype who is also closely associated with the in utero stage of life; in fact, she is the womb of sleep in which we can incubate our greatest potential. In the texts, she is described as deeply affectionate, and the one who gives us spiritual power and the capacity to hold the hazards of night at bay.

When we begin to use sleep as a method of accessing higher states of consciousness, we find that we have truly come into contact with the power that this great goddess represents. Yoga Nidra symbolizes what can occur when we awaken to a state of bliss that is our true nature. This changes how we experience all of life. We move beyond the physical body and conscious mind, and we start to connect to our ultimate source, consciousness. The state that we achieve when we are connected to this goddess is an aspect of pratyahara, which can lead to higher states of concentration and ultimately to *samadhi*. *Pratyahara* is a Sanskrit word meaning "withdrawal of the senses." *Samadhi* is a state of intense meditative awareness that allows us to experience union with our divine nature—in other words, enlightenment. Many of the ancient sages understood that there is an inherent mystical quality connected with sleep that allows us to withdraw our senses from the external distractions and connect with higher consciousness.

Throughout this book, we have offered many concrete examples of how awakened sleep can aid in optimal well-being. However, the gaps that science cannot fill have been explained by ancients across the globe, including those who compiled stories about Yoga Nidra. Many of these sages recorded the myths and teachings about the divine properties of sleep. Prophets from a variety of traditions received visions during dreams and other altered states. The births of Krishna, Buddha, and Jesus were all prophesied in dreams. A number of inventors, musicians, scientists, and other illustrious minds were specifically inspired after awakening from a vivid dream or a deep slumber, wherein they had greater access to their intuition, creativity, and higher states of consciousness, as we learned in the previous chapter. The ancient Vedas suggest a fine line between sleep, meditation, and enlightenment. Many of the teachings decode aspects of sleep, including dreams and other states of meditative awareness that we have yet to understand or integrate into our modern understanding of a higher or universal consciousness.

Sleep also has a correlation with the higher chakras, the junctions between matter and consciousness. The pineal gland, which corresponds to the crown chakra, is closely connected to divine consciousness, and is also the gland that secretes melatonin, the hormone that regulates our circadian rhythms and many other self-healing mechanisms in the body.

The pituitary gland and hypothalamus correspond to the third-eye chakra (the chakra that connects us to our intuition). The pea-sized pituitary gland is known as the master gland that is in charge of vital functions, including metabolism, growth, reproduction, and blood pressure. The pituitary gland also helps regulate sleep and the stress response. Along with the pituitary gland, the hypothalamus regulates the endocrine system and the intricate system of messenger molecules that flow throughout the body. The hypothalamus is also tied to the homeostatic sleep drive, which is the sense of pressure we feel driving us toward sleep.

Altogether, the higher chakras are also closely tied to the key functions of the higher brain, the cerebral cortex, which is the outermost layer of the brain. The cerebral cortex is responsible for the experience of pure awareness, and it plays a pivotal role in attention, memory, language, and spiritual awakening.

Researchers at Oxford, Yale, and Columbia universities discovered that spirituality-related activity largely resides in the part of the cerebral cortex known as the parietal cortex, the area of the brain that is most tied to our capacity for attention.[1] The researchers discovered that when their test subjects, each of whom shared that they'd had a spiritual awakening, recounted their experience, the neurological pattern was the same across all subjects; that is, activity was revealed in the parietal cortex. Amazingly, there was less activity in the left inferior parietal lobe, the part of the brain tied to awareness of self and others, and reduced activity in the medial thalamus and caudate, parts of the brain that process sensory input and emotions. The researchers concluded that in a spiritual awakening, when union with the divine is complete, there is loss of the sense of "I" and "you"—since people are no longer ruled by their egos but have melted into the absolute. Moreover, this is not a sensory or "emotional" experience. Similar to deep sleep, spiritual awakening is related to a withdrawal of the mind and senses altogether.

It's remarkable that modern science is beginning to reflect some of the concepts in Vedic philosophy, which equate sense withdrawal and merging with the absolute to the experience of enlightenment—as well as to the emergence of sattvic sleep, which we discussed in previous chapters. Ancient spiritual texts may also hold the key to the deeper meaning of sleep: what it does beyond merely regulating the functions of the mind and body, and how it can transform our experience as infinite beings in a finite form.

Going forward, we'll share some key aspects of what the ancients knew, as well as what science is beginning to tell us about our access to higher states of consciousness—and thus, to a spiritual well-being that can filter into our daily lives and create what some might consider miracles. Meditation invites us to slip into the hidden spaces of awareness, revealing deeper layers of reality—and with practice, we can even train ourselves to tap into this wisdom while we sleep.

ACCESS CONSCIOUSNESS WITH YOGA NIDRA

We've discussed the goddess known as Yoga Nidra, but you've probably heard this term being used to describe a popular form of guided meditation whose roots can be traced back to 700–1000 BCE. While previous chapters described various stages of sleep, yoga nidra itself tends to exist in the more liminal regions—in the hypnagogic state that people experience before falling asleep, and the hypnopompic state that occurs in the moments after waking up. In such a state, one isn't asleep, but one is not fully awake either. In this place, where the veils between our perception of "waking" reality and the ocean of consciousness are thin, we have a powerful opportunity to know our true selves.

As opposed to falling asleep, the intention of yoga nidra is to achieve a profound state of relaxation while maintaining awareness. The practice of yoga nidra, and this deep state of relaxation, has been shown to have a number of benefits. Many yogis have referred to it as a powerful psycho-spiritual healing technique that brings about altered states of consciousness through total physical and mental relaxation. As we begin to detach from the normal sensory channels, we connect with the true self—the part of us that is eternal and changeless, also referred to as atman.

Swami Satyananda Saraswati, who is credited with bringing yoga nidra into the mainstream in the 1960s, believed that the practice of placing our mind on a single point of focus has significant effects on the body. According to Swami Saraswati, yoga nidra is a state in which the entire body is infused with electromagnetic pulsations and vibrations. In such a state, the heart rate gradually slows and people become less susceptible to pain, to the extent that all tensions and discomforts in the body melt away. Yoga nidra also helps the practitioner to tap into interoception, a bodily sense that enables us to feel and decipher what is happening inside the body—which makes it easier to self-regulate, and also to expand into states that transcend the senses altogether.

Through a simple process of progressive relaxation, practitioners can experience a state of physical surrender accompanied by total mental awareness. Yoga nidra specifically works through the autonomic nervous system, which regulates the involuntary processes of the body—those processes that occur without our conscious effort. These include our heartbeat, breathing, digestion, and blood flow and encompass the sympathetic and parasympathetic nervous systems. In this state of deep relaxation, our immunity, digestion, and stress management are balanced. One study at the University of Tel Aviv discovered that yoga nidra may significantly lower levels of serum cholesterol in cardiac patients.[2] In fact, the link between yogic relaxation and the prevention of various forms of heart disease has been recognized for decades. Yoga nidra has also been shown to positively influence stress levels in the body, and according to a study from the National Institutes of Health, may be slightly more beneficial in reducing anxiety than meditation.[3] As the study notes, this may have a lot to do with the fact that the conscious mind is slowly guided to let go, making it easier to journey into the subconscious mind, which is not beleaguered by the same concerns that may be flitting around in our disorganized and distracted "waking" awareness—which can also make meditation difficult, especially for those who are managing acute anxiety.

Many people have used yoga nidra for a range of purposes. And although the term implies that it can improve sleep (which it absolutely does), the benefits also include healing physical or mental disorders and experiencing a greater receptivity to higher states of consciousness. A study that looked at the practice of yoga nidra in adolescents ages thirteen to fifteen showed improvement in multiple dimensions of well-being, including improvements in feelings of happiness, alertness, clarity of thought, and control over anger.[4] Some sleep researchers theorize that the natural states associated with yoga nidra, such as hypnagogia and dream states, can help us process and consolidate past experiences and prepare us for the future.[5]

There are various ways to practice yoga nidra. A form of yoga nidra known as iRest Yoga Nidra Meditation was developed by Dr. Richard Miller over a decade ago. Pilot studies have demonstrated that it can improve symptoms of stress and depression. It's also been used in the US military and veteran populations to treat PTSD, anxiety, pain, and sleep problems. In the modern context, variations on yoga nidra practices, as well as other types of relaxation practices, are referred to as *non-sleep deep rest*, or NSDR, a term coined by researcher and neuroscientist Dr. Andrew Huberman. These modern takes on an ancient practice recognize the profound benefits of breathing, visualization, and focused attention on the brain and nervous system.

Practicing yoga nidra requires getting into a supine position, although in some cases it can be done while sitting, and listening to a guide who takes you through a series of steps. At some point, as you relax into the body, you become drowsy, but due to the guiding voice, you don't fall fully asleep. The general experience of yoga nidra involves slowing down to the point of accessing the delta brainwave state. In this state, the body and mind rest, as in sleep, yet the practitioner is wide-awake. This state is considered to be most conducive to deep healing. Here, you enter the hypnagogic state, where the mind goes in and out of awareness, riding the wave between sleep and wakefulness. Yoga nidra extends this stage of early sleep, which usually only lasts a few minutes.

The purpose of yoga nidra is to get into a deep state of relaxation while also being engaged with what is happening so that you can maintain a conscious state of relaxed awareness. Some may experience myoclonic jerks, which involve the bodily sensation of falling. However, this can facilitate the release of stress in the body, much like meditation does— and when relaxed into, it can allow us to expand our awareness of higher realms.

Many people experience various sensory experiences, such as sounds, voices, and visions, or even a sense of being touched during the practice. Although in modern sleep science, the experiences that we have in this hypnagogic state are considered hallucinations or pathologies, from the Vedic perspective we are accessing the field of consciousness and have experiences outside of the familiar waking state. We awaken our inner senses and awareness. In doing so, we awaken the capacity to heal.

Yoga nidra is an important practice in awakened sleep, because it can activate our ability to witness the wave of rising and falling consciousness at all times in our life. How is this important when it comes to attaining mystical and meditative levels of awareness? As we become aware of the rising and falling wave of consciousness, we can start to watch as the structures of the one we call "me" subside. We become observers of our own thought processes. Being in this liminal state places us at the threshold of the conscious and unconscious mind, the place where we experience waking dreams. Yoga nidra helps us become much more aware of this in-between state in ways that prepare us for higher levels of consciousness and take us toward the possibility of samadhi, a return to our truest nature.

To prepare yourself for yoga nidra, you can practice doing a body scan at various points of the day. This is a mindfulness practice that includes taking time to scan your body, from head to toe, to check for areas of pain, tension, or discomfort—or to simply observe yourself. It's a great way to get into the habit of developing your interoception, and it's also been shown to improve sleep, reduce pain and anxiety, and contribute to a greater sense of self-compassion. Getting into a habit of regular body scans will prepare you for the "waking dream" practice of yoga nidra.

A basic yoga nidra routine usually looks like this:

1. Set a clear intention for your practice, perhaps a peaceful rest.
2. Trust that this practice will guide you into surrender while the part of you always observing from a place of higher consciousness holds you in the process.
3. Gently scan your body, releasing any tension that may hinder your access to deeper states of awareness.
4. Bring your focus to your breath, slowing it down into deep, rhythmic inhalations and exhalations.
5. Allow any emotions to arise, simply noticing them as they come and go.
6. Observe the flow of your thoughts without judgment—neither suppressing nor getting caught up in them—just witnessing them as they pass. Witness the stories your mind creates, recognizing them as part of the ego, not your true essence.

7. As you relax further, you are guided to place attention on various parts of the body one by one, both on the right and left sides of the body. Notice the sensations in each of these parts as you bring awareness there.

8. You are then led through internal visualizations of different images that you bring into awareness. You witness each image and release any labels or judgments related to the image. Simply witness.

9. Engage in a moment of conscious self-reflection, being fully present and aware, integrating your experience into your being.

10. Deepening the breath and moving slowly, you end the practice.

Throughout this entire practice, you might be drifting in and out of sleep. Some people end up falling asleep altogether while doing this practice, which is fine, but one of the great benefits of yoga nidra is that it allows us to harness our capacity to move consciously and smoothly from waking to sleeping and back. In other words, we hone our capacity to remain conscious of where we are from moment to moment, which can benefit us in all aspects of our lives. After all, the notion that our earthly existence is separate from our spiritual existence is dispelled by a practice like yoga nidra, which helps us ride the wave of unfolding awareness and move beyond simplistic dualities.

Although yoga nidra asks us to scan the body and focus on things like the right foot and the left foot, staying with the practice enables us to transcend the limitations of concepts like "left" and "right" altogether. We get to experience the dissolution of seemingly opposing pairs. We move beyond the realm of material phenomena and into subtler aspects of reality.

Dr. Sheila's patient Sara, a dynamic woman in her sixties, had always been the classic busy person, but she discovered that yoga nidra was the perfect way to slow down. A successful architect, she spent decades juggling the demands of her career, family, and personal life. Meditation was something she had dabbled in since her thirties, but it had always been a challenge. Despite trying various methods to calm her mind, nothing seemed to truly stick.

After studying at the Chopra Center, Sara became a regular meditator and incorporated yoga into her routine. She had a successful career and felt meaning and purpose. But life, as it does, threw challenges her way. Her husband of thirty-five years was diagnosed with a brain tumor during the pandemic, throwing their lives into chaos. The stress of managing his health, navigating her career, and being there for her kids and grandchildren during such a trying time left Sara utterly wiped out. Despite seeking therapy and trying countless methods for better sleep, she continued to struggle with insomnia and a restless mind.

Her therapist recommended guided meditations, which led her to explore a variety of practices on her meditation apps. While some offered temporary relief, Sara still found herself awake in the middle of the night, tangled in stressful thoughts. Then, one day, while searching for something new, she stumbled upon yoga nidra.

At first, Sara wasn't sure what to expect. She was still working part time and taking on the role of primary caregiver for her husband, so adding another practice to her already full schedule seemed daunting. But she decided to dive in, committing to yoga nidra every day. And slowly but surely, Sara began to notice something extraordinary.

While her sleep didn't improve immediately, she noticed a sharper mind and an unexpected sense of clarity. The stress that once clouded her thoughts seemed to dissipate, and she felt less mentally fatigued, despite still struggling with poor sleep. Intrigued, Sara spoke with others who were experiencing similar stress and discovered that yoga nidra had been used effectively in treating PTSD. Being an inquisitive Pitta type, she dove into research and was pleased to discover that yoga nidra was evidence based, with powerful benefits for the nervous system and brain.

She began to introduce yoga nidra into her evening routine before bed and extended her practice to fifteen minutes or longer. Although she still occasionally wakes up between 2 and 3 a.m., her approach to sleep has shifted. Instead of stressing over falling asleep, Sara focuses on deep relaxation, trusting that the rest will follow.

What also contributed to her healing was a blend of practices to support her overall wellness. During times of high stress, Sara added pranayama (breathing exercises) into her yoga routine. Ayurveda played a crucial role, too; understanding her Pitta nature helped Sara make mindful nutritious choices, ensuring she wasn't aggravating her body with the wrong foods, especially at night.

Sara's journey with yoga nidra has now expanded beyond her own practice. She shares its transformative effects with her friends, clients, and colleagues, encouraging them to embrace this powerful technique. Although her sleep isn't perfect, her mind is clearer, her stress levels have significantly reduced, and her brain and body are healing. Her adventures in exploring the liminal spaces of yoga nidra capture the very essence of awakened sleep.

To access an in-depth yoga nidra audio meditation, visit www.awakenedsleep.net. We recommend that you engage in this practice in lieu of your regular nighttime meditation or as an addition to it; we provide some guidance on how to do this in Chapter 10, where we discuss how you can create your own nighttime ritual for sleep.

Shavasana (Corpse Pose)

The yogic pose known as shavasana, or corpse pose, is a state of absolute relaxation that is necessary to master if we wish to access consciousness. We refer to it as *corpse pose* because the physical body is absolutely still. In shavasana, you are in a supine resting pose, flat on your back, with your arms and legs in a state of surrender, eyes closed, palms face up. It is a pose of complete surrender, and many yogis refer to it as the most advanced asana in all of yoga.

In this pose, we are able to experience ourselves in a pure, soulful state of watching and witnessing the tides of our breath and our awareness. Often, people who go into shavasana at the end of a yoga practice might be lying there for just a few moments before slipping into a state of relaxation. (You've probably been at a yoga class where you heard someone snoring because they were able to drop into that place rather immediately!)

The fifteenth-century text known as the *Hatha Yoga Pradipika* mentions that shavasana has a purifying quality to it. Today, we understand that being in this pose is adaptogenic, meaning it can calm our nervous system and regulate our stress response, and thus plunges us into a blissful state. Shavasana is usually the pose that one takes on during a yoga nidra practice because of its potential for launching us into the most profound meditative states.

Certainly, the notion of being in a "corpse" pose might sound intimidating, but it's a powerful practice to die to our limited human egos on a daily basis so that we can step more wholeheartedly into our more expanded self. With such an ego death, we can begin to see reality as it truly is. In this place, cravings and aversions disappear, and we get to experience the mysteries of the cycles of life—of creation itself as it rises and falls away. When we practice being with this, we understand that the identities we carry in the world will come and go. As we practice dissolving the ego and stepping into the pure, undying self, we develop the kind of fearlessness that will allow us to face our actual physical death with gentle courage.

QUANTUM SLEEP: TRANSCEND ILLUSIONS, EMBRACE ENLIGHTENMENT

Awakened sleep is not only the key to optimal well-being—it is also one of the greatest tools at our disposal when it comes to realizing our spiritual nature and experiencing enlightenment within our waking human reality. Sleep can be viewed as the key to enlightenment, as it uncovers the many perceptual limitations that might keep us from seeing ourselves as we are.

There are two specific ideas in Vedic philosophy that help us understand the role sleep can play in enlightenment: the five sheaths and the four states of consciousness.

The Five Sheaths

In Vedic philosophy, there are five *koshas* (which literally translates to "sheaths") that serve as barriers to our true self. The spiritual journey is the process of peeling away the koshas to discover who we truly are. The Vedas provide a powerful pathway to self-discovery that enables us to systematically uncover the five koshas.

The first kosha is the physical body, or *annamayakosha*, literally the body made of food. This encompasses all aspects of the material body, including bones, skin, muscles, connective tissue, fat, and the three doshas. A sense of poor health signals an imbalance in this kosha, and working with the principles of Ayurveda and balancing our physical body with the right diet and lifestyle (and sleep!) can bring us back into a state of equilibrium.

The second kosha is the energy body, *pranamayakosha*. This is connected to the movement of breath and electrical impulses in the body. When we experience problems with our respiration, as well as blockages in the chakras, we are experiencing an imbalance in this kosha. Practicing pranayama (breath awareness) can bring about balance here.

The next layer is the mental body, or *manomayakosha*, which involves our mind, including our thoughts and feelings. Lack of awareness signals an imbalance in this kosha, while practicing meditation, yoga nidra, and pratyahara (withdrawal of the senses) can balance us out.

Then, we come to the wisdom body, *vijnanamayakosha*, which is our intellect and intuition. If we feel that we do not have clarity of thought, we are likely encountering a blockage or imbalance here; practices like *dharana* (concentration), *dhyana* (inward focus), and learning to trust our intuition can balance this kosha.

Finally, we come to the bliss body, *anandamayakosha*, which is the aspect of our true self that enables us to experience our wholeness and our connection to all beings. It also includes the karmic body—the subtle vibration that contains the energetic imprint of our past lives, and our presence throughout time and space. Some might refer to it as the individual human soul. Imbalance in this kosha can feel like a disconnection or lack of meaning in life. We experience a sense of balance by continuing to engage in practices that bring us into a clear awareness of our true nature at all times.

For all its brilliance, the bliss body is still also a sheath (albeit the thinnest one) that covers our true self. All the practices connected to awakened sleep help us peel past the layers and limitations of the koshas. We recognize that we are not ultimately our physical body, our energy body, our mental body, our wisdom body, or even our bliss body: We are consciousness itself. Awakened sleep helps us realize that the ocean of consciousness is bottomless, and when we merge with it, we experience an ego death that helps us move past the preoccupations of the mind (which is what most of our dreams tend to be generated from). In awakened sleep, we discover that, unmoored from our ideas of the ego-bound self, we can literally go anywhere and experience anything. In fact, with awakened sleep, we can transcend the waking and dreaming states altogether to experience enlightenment.

As we've shared in previous chapters, awakened sleep is sattvic sleep—the sleep that is infused with the qualities of absolute serenity, peace, and love. Although we might not necessarily have the experience of merging with the ocean of consciousness 24/7 in our waking lives, we can still carry the quality of awakened sleep into our daily encounters. That is, we can enjoy sensory pleasures while remaining unattached to them; we can experience conflict without being sucked into it; we can be passionate about our specific contribution to the world while recognizing the true self beyond any role we play. Awakened sleep makes it possible to be in touch with the field of the absolute and eternal at all times.

The Four States of Consciousness

The *Upanishads* detail the four states of consciousness; specifically, the *Mandukya Upanishad* describes these states as waking, dreaming, deep sleep, and *turiya* (the state of pure witnessing awareness). Awakened sleep allows us to integrate all these different states of consciousness— even making it possible to bring the fruits of turiya back into our waking state.

In our waking state, the atman (the soul, or spirit) is typically forgotten as we come to identify almost entirely with the physical body (the first kosha). This is the most illusory and limited state of awareness. We ourselves identify as a sensory object rather than identifying with consciousness. We are limited by the rules of the material world. As we become caught up in sensory experiences, cravings, and aversions that keep us stuck in a mental and emotional tug-of-war, we can lose sight of the spiritual self.

In our dreaming state, we identify with the second and third koshas: the energy body and the mental body—especially when we are journeying through dreams that kick up the thoughts and emotions of our daily lives. Dream state is considered a projection of the mind. Sometimes we merge with our wisdom body, or intellect, in the instances when we have dreams that illuminate different perspectives and understandings of our experiences. Such dreams could include powerful symbols (such as guides, angels, or deities) or even moments of lucidity when we begin to realize that we are dreaming.

In deep sleep, we merge with the bliss body. Deep sleep is the absence of experience, or one could say the experience of absence. Here, we are free of the perception of external objects or internal thoughts (including the object of "self"), and the mind is quiet. In deep sleep we are as close to accessing consciousness as we are during meditation, and it gives us a glimpse of the true nature of consciousness, which is why it is so restorative. However, as it is a complete absence of external awareness, it is also a temporary state of unconsciousness.

Finally, in turiya, we no longer identify with the koshas. We are awareness being aware of itself. We are beyond the states of waking, dreaming, and deep sleep. This is true witnessing of awareness. Our ignorance and misperceptions disappear as we begin to realize who we truly are. All the worlds we have previously navigated appear to be a dream. As we cultivate this transcendence, we can begin to experience awareness even in deep sleep.

After this state, we experience samadhi: total absorption into the ultimate reality. This isn't considered to be one of the four states of consciousness, because it transcends all experience, and even awareness itself. We connect completely to the witness within, and there is no longer a sense of "I." We have finally merged with the ocean of consciousness and feel a sense of oneness with the universe.

Awakened sleep ultimately helps us connect to this inner witness, but we must prepare ourselves for this process. We cannot be an enlightened yogi at night and a human bogged down in the stuff of our daily physical reality during the day. Awakened sleep begins in our waking hours, when we do what is necessary to program, regulate, and modulate the mind so that we move from contracted to expanded states of consciousness. Awakened sleep also helps us return to our waking reality while remaining in that expanded state of divine flow. We will have the experience of all our true needs being effortlessly met, because we have removed the obstacles that get in the way. In our sleep, our unconscious mind has worked to polish and refine our awareness, so that there is no debris left to be sorted out in our dreams. Thus, the tide of dream and deep sleep can move us into the realm of turiya, where we transcend the illusions of maya, a.k.a. reality as we know it.

If any of this sounds unattainable, remember that it isn't. Self-realization is a feature, not a bug, of our design. One doesn't have to be a super yogi to attain sense withdrawal; we can do this naturally when we sleep, which allows for the possibility of disidentifying from the body and the mind. While many of us still experience the residue of the energy and mental bodies while we slumber, awakened sleep helps us go several steps beyond until the subject-object split is gone altogether. Deep relaxation makes it possible for the distinction between "me" and "that" to disappear, even if it's for only the shortest period of time. As we move into the bliss body (which is possible in deep sleep), we can even begin burning away our accumulated karmas (also known as *samskaras*, which are the accumulated energetic patterns and mental impressions that rule our habits and what we carry from lifetime to lifetime).

With this, we start to effortlessly minimize our obstacles toward enlightenment—obstacles that might include addictive behaviors, difficult relationship patterns, and low self-worth. This is why, throughout Vedic texts, sleep is recognized as a terminal state that can take us well past our limitations and habitual patterns and into new possibilities. The outcome of awakened sleep, as in meditation, is self-regulation toward our natural state of health and happiness.

We've noticed that with the journey into awakened sleep, many people who might have been inconsistent with a spiritual or meditative practice are able to integrate these activities into their lives with greater ease and joy. As they tap into consciousness, the realm of infinite creativity through awakened sleep, many have the experience of receiving mystical downloads, such as music or even an entire book; they are then inspired to share this creativity with the world. Our lives become more creative and filled with greater synchronicities (meaningful occurrences that cannot be chalked up to mere coincidence). We are able to get into a "thoughtless" state more easily, where we are simply entering and flowing with life as if we were partaking in a beautiful dance whose steps we innately know, even if we haven't been through them before. Instead of using our past thoughts and experiences as references, we approach each moment as a new opportunity.

And although we can instill habits that help us move closer to our true nature, we must not be too attached to the idea of how that's supposed to look. We need not try to achieve states like lucidity in our dreams, or awareness of the bliss body, or samadhi. The more we relax and detach from our expectations, the easier it will become to find what we seek. We will also see tangible changes in our own life, to the extent that nirvana, or self-realization, becomes the all-pervasive experience we have, whether we're asleep or awake.

Living in this state of transcendental awareness may sound like it requires living on a mountain, away from the cares of our daily reality, but this isn't the case. The more we engage with practices of awakened sleep, the more capable we become of integrating our mystical experiences into our everyday lives. This is why meditation is of such great benefit to us—because it gets us into the practice of "finding the gap" in our experience and stepping into a nonjudgmental witnessing role. We become less reactive, and it gets easier to access states of peace, harmony, love, and compassion, no matter what the circumstances of our life might be. We begin to experience this awakened consciousness in ourselves, and then we see it in everything and everyone around us.

The purpose of awakened sleep is to bring that transcendent consciousness into our daily lives and interactions. It's a lot like dipping a garment into a vat of dye over time. The more we do it, the more the color seeps into the fabric. Just like that, the more we engage with awakened sleep, the more we transform over time. We might still play the part of a spouse, parent, student, entrepreneur, or any number of roles in our daily life, but we become more and more connected to who we truly are, and this heals us on a cellular level, unlike anything else can.

Vasant, Dr. Suhas's father-in-law, struggled with insomnia for decades. In the last twenty years, Vasant adopted a technique known as *brahmavidya*, an ancient practice that combines meditation and specialized breathing techniques. He gradually got to a point where he could sleep roughly 3.5 hours a night, without any sleep medication, and wake up feeling perfectly energized. He's eighty-nine years old and is in robust health. He's as sharp as a razor and can easily recall events that happened decades ago. At first, Dr. Suhas felt that Vasant's "sleep debt" would come back to haunt him later in his life. In fact, research has shown that if you lose sleep over time, full recovery to optimal health can be challenging. However, through meditation and a healthy lifestyle, Vasant has created awakened sleep in his life.

All of this ties back to Chapter 1 and our discussion about well-being. When we begin to tap into awakened sleep, seemingly unorthodox ways of sleeping (e.g., getting only a few hours of sleep at night, sleeping with noise or in a challenging environment, etc.) can allow us to tap into a powerful source of well-being. Most medical recommendations are based on getting people back to a neutral baseline (which is why we always hear about the requisite eight hours of sleep), but awakened sleep asks us not to settle for neutral. Awakened sleep allows us to go beyond neutral and to thrive in all aspects of our lives. Experiencing it means that we still follow commonsense guidelines—but there may be cases when we throw out the rules and awaken to a deep, restorative sense of well-being that takes us way beyond good sleep.

Heart Chakra Meditation

Simply focusing attention on the heart has been shown to calm the nervous system and reduce inflammation in the body. We teach our patients a meditative practice they can do in the evening a few hours before bed; it involves focusing on the heart while silently repeating a sound, or mantra. Patients can also use any other form of mantra-based meditation technique, which similarly aids in a sense of inner calm and deep relaxation. The mantra syncs with the nervous system and takes us into a deep state of awareness that further cultivates our capacity for awakened sleep.

As we mentioned in Chapter 5, mantra, as a primordial sound, is related to the element of space. In fact, *nada brahma* is a term that refers to "the sound of god," as sound is thought to be a fundamental aspect of the creation of the universe in Vedic philosophy. Thus, mantra can be used to literally take us to the space of creation, which transcends the boundaries of the physical body. With it, we are no longer in danger of falling into the slumber of tamas—the sleep of darkness and ignorance.

As we meditate, we focus on the heart chakra, which connects the higher three chakras with the lower three. The heart is a junction point, the space between our cosmic self and our earthly instinctive self. It can be seen as the gateway to transcendent states of consciousness.

Organizations like the HeartMath Institute have studied the extraordinary benefits of meditating while focused on the heart. We know that the heart has the largest, most powerful electromagnetic field in the body—sixty times greater than that of the brain. In the 1990s, researchers at the HeartMath Institute identified something they refer to as *heart coherence*, which occurs when all the systems of the body (circulatory, respiratory, hormonal, nervous system, etc.) are in sync.[6] They went on to develop techniques that help us shift out of the head and into the heart for greater peace and well-being.

In Ayurveda, the heart is the place where *ojas* and *tejas* are generated. Ojas is the vital essence that is the healthy end product of digesting our food and life experience. When it's in abundance, we have good immunity and a high level of happiness. Without it, we feel depressed, lethargic, and weak. The word *tejas* literally translates to "fire" or "illumination" and is an energy associated with both vitality and love. When we focus our awareness on the heart with one-pointed attention, ojas and tejas flow in greater quantities, our immune system is optimized, and our nervous system is regulated.

Below is a simple nighttime technique you can try for awakened sleep. We have a more extensive awakened sleep meditation you can try right before bedtime (which you'll find in Chapter 10); you can do this one before bedtime, but it can also be done at the sattvic hour of sunset, roughly around 6 p.m.

1. Sit in an upright posture, with support for your back if needed. If you are doing this meditation before bedtime, lie down on your back with a light pillow supporting your head.
2. Become aware of your breathing. Breathe smoothly and evenly, without any pause or sound.
3. Take time to quickly scan your body from head to toe, using your breath and attention to relax any areas of tension or discomfort.
4. Once you feel sufficiently relaxed, bring attention to the region around your heart. Allow a sense of appreciation, compassion, love, or gratitude into this area.
5. After a few moments, begin reciting the mantra *Om Shanti. Om* is the syllable that denotes the primordial sound of creation, and

shanti relates to a state of restful awareness, peace, and love. You can also use any personalized mantra you have received.

6. With every exhalation, repeat your mantra. With every inhalation, focus your attention on the area around your heart, noticing the warm flow of tejas and ojas and the sense of peace and quietude this brings. This circulating awareness is effortlessly connected with the greater field of consciousness that is helping you transcend the boundaries of your physical body and connect with your true self and infinite potential.

7. After five to ten minutes, stop reciting the mantra and simply let it vibrate deeply in your heart and slowly open your eyes.

As you rest in this awareness, you will move into the remainder of your day in a state of open-hearted calm; if you're doing it before bedtime, keep your eyes closed and you will slowly drift into a state of awakened sleep.

EMBRACE THE UNKNOWN

We recently spoke with a forty-seven-year-old woman named Nicky who works in a demanding job in the sales industry. She was on an Ayurvedic regimen to manage infertility, and she'd begun to adopt a regimen of daily meditation that was helping her improve her sleep. One evening, she was feeling anxious about having to fire one of her employees the following morning. However, she focused on relaxing her body and melting away any residual stress with her meditation practice. She went to bed that night and had an extraordinary experience: While she was sleeping, she'd somehow mapped out an entire script for what she would say to the employee. She was also able to hear his responses in detail. They had a constructive and easy conversation in the dream that helped her prepare for the events of the following day.

Amazingly, when Nicky went into work that morning, the conversation she had with the employee went exactly the way it had in her dream, down to every last word! It was almost as if she'd gone through a dress rehearsal in her sleep, and she'd been shown the way she should enter the conversation. Rather than it being stressful, she was able to eliminate any negativity or judgment from the conversation. The result was an honest and thoughtful exchange that made both her and the employee feel a sense of relief and positive anticipation for what was next.

Nicky felt proud of herself for surrendering the situation to a greater possibility and awareness—a higher, more expansive way of communicating with her employee. Rather than attempting to problem-solve with her conscious mind, she trusted that withdrawing her senses and connecting with cosmic intelligence and the field of potentiality would enable her to see the big picture and determine the best way to approach the situation. This also helped her detach from the outcome and be less reactive during the conversation. It was almost as if Nicky's sleep state had helped her transcend her egoic limitations and tap into a greater field of knowledge and awareness that allowed her to act in a way that was beneficial for everyone involved.

Science is still beginning to put the pieces together as to how exactly this works, but there is a growing field of inquiry in neuroscience that's known as *nonlocal consciousness*. According to this theory, the mind and consciousness itself don't exist inside the brain. Rather, it is everywhere and nowhere all at once. Some suggest that it is also not time bound. That is, when we tap into nonlocal consciousness, we might interface with past memories, present experiences, and future possibilities. So, it could be that Nicky's "dress rehearsal" was just a future possibility presenting itself to her, so that she could step into it in her waking life.

In our waking lives, time and space are part of the great illusion that we experience in our earthbound reality. Of course, this illusion may continue to captivate us to some extent, but it's also possible to break out of it now and then, especially as we continue to experiment within the mystical realm of awakened sleep.

REFLECTIONS

1. What are you most curious about when it comes to exploring consciousness? Have you noticed moments of heightened awareness or altered states that left a lasting impression?
2. Reflect on your relationship with spiritual well-being. How has prioritizing this area influenced your daily life, health, and sleep quality?
3. Practice the yoga nidra meditation on pages 211–212 three times before bedtime. How does your body respond during the meditation? What do you notice in your mind, and how does this practice influence your sleep experience?
4. Reflect on any shifts in awareness or mental clarity that you notice during or after meditation. How does this affect your sense of restfulness and inner peace?
5. As you prepare to design a personalized sleep-hygiene protocol in Part 3, what aspects of consciousness and meditation would you like to integrate into your nightly routine? What practices do you feel drawn to explore further?

List any takeaways from this chapter that you'd like to incorporate into your own sleep-hygiene routine:

_____

_____

_____

_____

_____

PART 3

REST FOR SUCCESS—CREATE
THE PERFECT ROUTINE
FOR AWAKENED SLEEP

CHAPTER 9

)) ● ((

ENERGIZE YOUR DAY—
MAKE THE MOST OF
YOUR SUNSHINE

*We sleep, but the loom of life never stops and the
pattern which was weaving when the sun went
down is weaving when it comes up tomorrow.*

—Henry Ward Beecher

BASED ON ALL THAT YOU'VE LEARNED SO FAR AS WELL AS ON YOUR responses to the assessments and reflection questions, we'll be exploring the power of establishing a daily routine that supports a lifestyle conducive to awakened sleep.

Now that you've learned about the physical, mental/emotional, and spiritual benefits of awakened sleep, it's time to incorporate this accumulated knowledge into your life. It is becoming increasingly recognized in medicine that personalization is needed when it comes to helping a person sleep.[1] After all, there's no such thing as one-size-fits-all—especially not in the realm of awakened sleep.

In this chapter, we'll cover the hours from 6 a.m. to 6 p.m., which make up the bulk of your day and the basis of your dinacharya (daily routine). *Dina* refers to the daytime, and *charya* to the idea of cycles. A dinacharya is a circular routine that enables you to train your mind, body, and internal clock to a series of precisely timed activities. The more disrupted this routine becomes, the more your circadian rhythm will be disrupted—which can lead to dosha imbalances and many of the chronic disorders and compromises to your overall well-being that we've discussed so far.

We cannot stress enough the importance of regularity. You're training your mind and body to establish a sense of balance throughout the day that prepares you for a night of sattvic, awakened sleep. We accumulate toxins when our life experiences aren't completely metabolized. An intentional daily routine focuses on detoxification, purification, and rejuvenation, so that we are keeping our physical and emotional digestive systems strong and clear—which contributes to awakened sleep. Our dinacharya essentially harmonizes our internal rhythms with those of nature, improving our capacity for daily self-renewal and our ability to go into our ratricharya (evening routine) with a palpable sense of calm and balance.

First, we'll explore a generalized Ayurvedic daytime routine, which encompasses all three doshas, as well as life stages and special considerations (e.g., shift workers, global travelers, new parents, and women going through menopause and perimenopause). This routine is the foundation for awakened sleep. It includes the six pillars of physical, mental/emotional, and spiritual well-being: stress management and meditation, emotional regulation, movement, nutrition, self-care, and sleep hygiene.

Next, we'll explore the ways in which you can tweak the general routine to your dosha (or dosha imbalance). Finally, we'll integrate all you've learned throughout the previous chapters; you will be supported to use the dosha clock and the various assessments and information you've gleaned from the reflection exercises to build a daytime routine that enables you to ease into and manage your day with greater clarity and awareness. We encourage you to deeply consider the power of conscious consumption (of everything from food to thoughts to stimuli) and will also offer some insight with respect to how you can customize the recommendations to your own circumstances and lifestyle.

While we encourage you to design a routine for yourself that follows closely with the foundational daytime routine we introduce in this chapter, we're fully aware that everyone's life circumstances are different. For example, you might currently be taking sleep medications, or perhaps your work schedule makes it impossible to wake up around sunrise. Please remember that even a few intentional (and regular!) additions to your daily routine can make a world of difference; you don't need to incorporate all of them right away. Awakened sleep is truly accessible to everyone, and we encourage you not to make perfection the enemy of good.

In addition, you may find that you go through seasonal shifts that require a slightly different daily routine (for example, waking up at 7 a.m. rather than 6 a.m. during the fall and winter seasons, and with daylight saving time). We aren't here to present you with rules but to share with you what works, based on thousands of years of Vedic wisdom. We encourage you to experiment with whatever fits your particular lifestyle while keeping our primary recommendations in mind. Also, revisit the breakout boxes, reflection questions, and assessments throughout the book for specific, detailed instructions on activities you might wish to incorporate into your morning routine—including breathwork, meditation, and journaling practices.

A FOUNDATIONAL DAYTIME ROUTINE

Between 6 and 10 a.m.

This is the Kapha time of day, associated with the elements of water and earth. It's cool (and usually damp) outside, and nature is just waking up. During this period, the body can feel dull and heavy. You may feel congested. Your digestion is still in the process of waking up. Although all these practices are part of an ideal morning routine, choose a few to start with and gradually add practices over time based on your own schedule. Make the ones that are the most nourishing part of your daily routine, and bring in the other practices when you can.

- Awaken at 6 a.m., without the accompaniment of an alarm clock, which can unnecessarily jar you out of sleep. (If you sleep past 6 a.m., moving further into Kapha time, you may end up feeling more sluggish; if you do wake up later, you can kick-start your body into motion with some exercise as movement will invigorate the heavy and slow qualities of Kapha.)
- Consider not turning on phones or tuning in to the news of the day until after your early-morning routine and the Kapha hours.
- If you remember any of your dreams from the previous night and you keep a record of them for the purpose of deeper emotional processing, briefly jot down your memories.
- Empty your bowels and bladder.
- Do oil pulling and tongue scraping before brushing your teeth.
- Thoroughly cleanse your eyes and face.
- Use nasya drops and/or a neti pot to clear out nasal congestion.

- Drink a glass of warm water with a few drops of lemon juice. Drink one glass of plain warm water, or rinse your mouth with warm water, afterward.
- Perform exercises depending on your needs (e.g., for flexibility, strength, or cardio—refer to the dosha specifications for types of exercise to choose).
- Expose yourself to morning sunlight, either by stepping outside or gazing out a window.
- Spend time in meditation. We recommend at least twenty to thirty minutes, if possible. Perform five minutes of a breathing technique, either before or after meditation.
- Massage your body with a warm oil.
- Bathe or shower.
- Eat a light seasonal breakfast, per your dosha type and hunger level.
- Perform your work and other morning activities with awareness.

Between 10 a.m. and 2 p.m.

From 10 a.m. onward, we move into the Pitta hours, associated with fire and water. This is the time when the sun is highest in the sky, and when both the mind and digestive system are at their most active. Pitta time is ideal for bringing your focus to any activities that require a sharp mind, focus, and critical thinking.

- Eat your biggest meal of the day between 12 noon and 1 p.m.
- Sit quietly for five minutes after eating and then go for a short walk, even if indoors.
- Continue to perform your afternoon work and activity.

- Take frequent breaks of one to two minutes to stand, stretch, or engage in deep breathing or eye exercises.

Between 2 and 6 p.m.

This is the time when Vata dominates. Vata, representing the elements of space and air, brings creativity and inspiration to our activities. If you've had a busy morning, you might find that you need to rest between different activities during this period.

- Continue to perform your afternoon work and activity.
- Consider journaling or performing some breathing to release any intense emotions or experiences of the day.
- Avoid caffeine after 3 p.m.
- Meditate in the late afternoon to early evening, between 4 and 6 p.m.
- Do any sports or cardio activity prior to dinner.
- Eat a light, seasonal dinner, per your dosha and digestive strength.
- Take a short, leisurely walk for five to ten minutes after dinner, or do another simple movement practice.

MODIFY YOUR ROUTINE FOR THE DOSHAS

Refer to the assessment from Chapter 1 (What Kind of Sleeper Are You?, page 40) to find your prakruti (the dosha or natural constitution with which you were born) and the assessment from Chapter 2 (Which Dosha Is Keeping You Up at Night?, page 70) to find your *vikruti* (your current imbalances). Then, based on both of these, check out the dosha-balancing tips below, which can be used to round out your daily routine.

Vata

- Favor warm food and drinks, such as warm soups and teas, over cold ones.
- Ensure that your meals are well cooked and easy to digest. Reduce raw or dry foods.
- Engage in light exercise. Vata-pacifying exercises include tai chi, gentle yoga, walking, short hikes, and light cycling.
- Use sesame or almond oil, and slow, light strokes in your self-massage practice.
- Dress to stay warm.
- Take brief naps in the late afternoon, during Vata time, when needed and avoid overscheduling your day.
- Engage in practices that are grounding—such as mindful breathing, mindful eating, gentle movement, "earthing" (the practice of connecting with the earth's natural energy by physically touching the ground, such as walking barefoot on grass, sand, or soil), short breaks in nature, etc.

Pitta

- Favor cooling food and drinks, such as fresh fruits and vegetables.
- Reduce acidic, salty, and spicy tastes.
- Use coconut or olive oil, and strong, deep strokes in your self-massage practice.
- Dress so that your body temperature remains cool.
- Engage in moderate exercise in the morning, such as brisk walking or jogging, biking, skiing, swimming, and

outdoor activities. Avoid overheating—and avoid being overly competitive!

- Avoid overdoing; create space in your schedule to decompress.
- Engage in practices that increase a sense of detachment and acceptance, such as gratitude practice, community service, guided visualization, etc.

Kapha

- Favor a light diet of warm, dry foods, such as salads and leafy greens. Stay away from heavy foods that cause congestion, such as meat and dairy products.
- Add spices to your diet to increase metabolism and digestion, such as cayenne, black pepper, ginger, etc.
- Instead of oil massage, try dry brushing to get energy moving; or use light oils for self-massage such as safflower or sunflower oils.
- Dress to stay warm.
- Partake in vigorous and longer workouts (thirty to forty minutes if possible), such as running, aerobics, dance, rowing, active yoga, and weight training.
- Engage in practices that increase a sense of both awareness and lightness, such as mindful eating, laughter yoga, listening to uplifting and energizing music, decluttering, etc.

REFLECTIONS

Compare your responses to the following questions to the foundational daytime routine in this chapter. Spend time with your responses and consider how you might be able to modify your current routine to create one that works for you and that provides a welcome window into awakened sleep.

1. When do you naturally wake up without the accompaniment of an alarm clock?
2. How often do you move your bowels, and when?
3. When do you eat your first meal of the day?
4. When do you eat your largest meal?
5. How often do you exercise?
6. Do you have a morning exercise routine? If so, what does it generally entail?
7. What time do you typically put away work and other gadgets to wind down your day?
8. How often do you quietly sit to check in with your mind and body?
9. Do you have a meditation practice? If so, what times do you meditate during the day? If not, what might be getting in the way?
10. Do you have a different schedule on weekends? If so, what is it?
11. Which of your doshas needs balancing now?
12. How are your environment and lifestyle contributing to your dosha balance?
13. Overall, are you nourishing your body, mind, and spirit daily?
14. And are you supporting all six pillars of your well-being throughout the day?

CRAFT YOUR OWN DAYTIME ROUTINE

Go back to the assessment in Chapter 3 (Your Dosha Clock—Time Your Perfect Day, page 102), which you can use as a reference to create a more comprehensive morning routine for your dosha. Pay attention to the way your general routine (whether it's regular or not) makes you feel. Can you commit to creating a routine that takes your dosha and potential dosha imbalances into account, which will increase the likelihood of experiencing restorative, awakened sleep? We hope you feel empowered to choose activities from our previous suggestions that fit each hour of the day. And if you're one of the many people who balks at the idea of structure, we encourage you to see this as an opportunity to embark on a brand-new adventure that prioritizes your well-being. Our patients who are initially reluctant to adopt a regular routine but try it on for size are always happy to report that they experience more energy, clarity, insight, and, of course, awakened sleep when they accept the reframe that a routine doesn't have to be boring or feel restrictive. In fact, it can free us up so that we experience well-being in all domains.

Before you create your own daily routine, based on what you've learned in this chapter and throughout the book, take a look at the following daily routine. Moira is one of our patients who travels at least twice a month. She is forty-eight years old with a primary Vata dosha (prakruti). She had experienced symptoms of menopause, with hot flashes and sleep disturbance, an expression of some accumulated Pitta imbalance. In addition to having an active, busy work life as a marketing professional, Moira has two kids, ages ten and fourteen. Moira makes a healthy, light breakfast for the whole family in the morning (during which they sit together, without smartphones, and discuss their positive intentions for the day), but now that her children are old enough to wake up on their own and move through their own routines, she is able to prioritize her early-morning self-care.

Time of Day	Dominant Dosha	Activities
6–7 a.m.	Kapha	Wake up between 6 and 6:30 a.m. Look out the window at the morning sky. Do some journaling on dreams I can remember as well as on intention-setting for the day. Empty bowels and bladder. Brush teeth, clean tongue. Wash face and eyes.
7–8 a.m.	Kapha	Take online gentle yoga class for thirty minutes (do this outdoors if it's warm enough, or close to a window). Meditate (paired with Breath of the Ocean from Chapter 6) for twenty minutes.
8–9 a.m.	Kapha	Perform a self-massage and take a shower. Eat breakfast (usually oatmeal or a warm soup, with a noncaffeinated tea) with kids and husband, where we share our gratitude and intentions for the day ahead.
9–10 a.m.	Kapha	Take a short, ten-minute walk around the neighborhood before settling into home office. Look at email and other messages and take time to mindfully, slowly respond to them. Set agenda for the day ahead, including travel plans.
10–11 a.m.	Pitta	Attend work meetings.
11 a.m.–12 noon	Pitta	Attend work meetings.
12 noon–1 p.m.	Pitta	Eat a nourishing vegetarian lunch (current favorites are kale and carrot soup with ginger, fennel, and lime; quinoa with vegetables; red lentil dal; an assortment of fruit). Take a fifteen-minute walk after lunch unless it's too cold or hot outside, then get steps indoors.
1–2 p.m.	Pitta	Attend work meetings.
2–3 p.m.	Vata	Perform more creative work (developing social media plans and templates, keynote presentations, working on the book that I'm writing, etc.).

Time of Day	Dominant Dosha	Activities
3–4 p.m.	Vata	Continue creative work, with stretch/breathing breaks.
4–5 p.m.	Vata	Continue creative work, with stretch/breathing breaks.
5–6 p.m.	Vata	Take a break to journal and meditate (Safe and Sound—an Emotional-Release Process from Chapter 6, Heart Chakra Meditation from Chapter 8). Do a twenty-minute calming yoga sequence online before connecting with family and starting dinner.

Now, it's time to create your own personalized routine from the suggestions in this chapter:

Time of Day	Dominant Dosha	Activities
6–7 a.m.	Kapha	
7–8 a.m.	Kapha	
8–9 a.m.	Kapha	
9–10 a.m.	Kapha	

Time of Day	Dominant Dosha	Activities
10–11 a.m.	Pitta	
11 a.m.–12 noon	Pitta	
12 noon–1 p.m.	Pitta	
1–2 p.m.	Pitta	
2–3 p.m.	Vata	
3–4 p.m.	Vata	
4–5 p.m.	Vata	
5–6 p.m.	Vata	

CHAPTER 10

)) ● ((

SOOTHED BY MOONLIGHT-CREATE YOUR EVENING RITUAL FOR AWAKENED SLEEP

There is a time for many words and
there is also a time for sleep.

—Homer, *The Odyssey*

NOW THAT YOU'VE CREATED YOUR OWN MORNING ROUTINE, WE'LL cover the basics of creating a foundational evening routine (ratricharya), from 6 p.m. and into your sleeping hours. Throughout, we've covered a great deal of ground on what it means to prepare a sanctuary for your sleep, internally and externally, so we encourage you to go back to the earlier chapters for specific instruction.

Here, we'll cover restorative techniques for relaxing your mind, body, and spirit prior to sleep. As we did in Chapter 9, we'll offer guidance that's pertinent to each dosha, but this chapter also includes an extended meditation for awakened sleep that anyone can do. The goal of this chapter is to help you pull weeds and plant seeds in the field of consciousness right before sleep, free of the distractions and sensory stimuli that often carry into the night. We especially encourage you to revisit Chapter 5 for some useful tips on making your bedroom your own special sanctuary and using five-senses therapy to prepare for awakened sleep.

A FOUNDATIONAL EVENING AND NIGHTTIME ROUTINE

- Eat a light to moderate dinner between 6 and 7 p.m. at the latest, at least two to three hours before sleep (avoid foods that are heavy, sticky, overly spicy, or difficult to digest and opt for cooked, warm, satiating food in quantities appropriate for your appetite).
- Sit quietly for five minutes after eating.
- Take a short walk (five to fifteen minutes) to aid in digestion if weather permits; otherwise, do some other movement in the house.
- Perform light activity that doesn't require expending too much mental or physical energy (e.g., knitting, reading, doing a puzzle, listening to a relaxing podcast, simple household chores, light conversation, etc.).
- Take a warm bath with your preferred soothing essential oil, or our suggested blend (lavender, rosemary, and orange, which balance all three doshas); you can also place these oils in an aromatherapy diffuser or place a few drops on your pillow.
- Perform a relaxing self-massage while preparing your bath, being sure to massage your fingers, toes, and soles of your feet.

- Wash your face thoroughly.
- Use ghee or eye drops to clear and moisturize your eyes. Do some eye exercises.
- Put a few drops of oil into each of your ears; plug your ears with a small cotton ball; alternatively, you can gently massage your ears with oil.
- If desired, drink a warm cup of herbal tea or golden milk with cardamom or nutmeg.
- Do oil pulling and tongue scraping before brushing your teeth.
- Perform gentle yoga stretches for ten to fifteen minutes.
- Change into loose-fitting sleepwear in cotton or silk.
- Cultivate peace and clarity by releasing negative emotions via journaling, or read uplifting literature.
- Keep your bedroom dark and at a temperature that feels good to you.
- Remove all screens from your bedroom.
- Set intentions before sleep (e.g., planting seeds for the kinds of dreams you'd like to have or the messages you'd like to program into your subconscious mind).
- For about twenty to thirty minutes, or however long it takes you, do the Awakened Sleep Technique (below), which integrates many of the meditative and breathwork practices we've offered throughout this book.
- Be in bed with the lights off no later than 10:30 p.m.

AWAKENED SLEEP TECHNIQUE

Our technique is meant to be a cumulative practice that increases its benefits over time. As you continue to do this technique, adding your own variations where you see fit, you will gradually train yourself to automatically shift into awakened sleep.

Phase 1: Prepare for the Journey

1. Turn off all the lights and rid the room of any ambient noise.

2. Sitting up in bed, look around and take in the total darkness with your eyes open. Let your breathing be normal and unhurried.

3. Now, close your eyes, sensing the darkness. Take several deep breaths.

4. Gently lie down on your back.

5. Keep your eyes closed and continue slow, rhythmic breathing, taking at least five seconds for each inhalation and exhalation.

6. Now, one by one, draw your attention to your sense organs and senses. Start with your ears/sound, move on to skin/touch, then eyes/sight, tongue/taste, and finally, nose/smell. Spend a few minutes on each sense before moving on to the next. Detach from any evaluation about what you are perceiving and simply witness.

7. Now pay attention to your mind and your thoughts, not holding on too tightly to anything that arrives in your awareness. Simply notice it and let it go.

8. After a few minutes, recapitulate and rewind through your entire day. Review everything you experienced, from the time you woke up all the way to the present moment. Try to stay in a place of just observing your day rather than judging or evaluating your experiences.

9. Express heartfelt feelings of joy and gratitude for yourself and everyone in your life, perhaps even including the difficulties that have contributed to your growth.

Phase 2: Enter the Womb of Creation*

1. Continuing with your eyes closed, bring your attention to your heart and notice your breath here. Simply notice the rise and fall of your chest as your breath comes naturally.

2. Feel the pulsation, vibration, and connect to the flow of prana (primal life force/subtle energy of air), tejas (inner radiance/subtle energy of fire), and ojas (primal vitality/subtle energy of water).

3. Now moving your awareness to the whole body, feel the warm, gentle flow of *soma* (the subtle nectar of truth, light, and bliss) that envelops you and circulates from head to toe.

4. Starting with the top of your head (or vice versa), relax your head and face.

5. Relax your neck and shoulders.

6. Relax your upper arms, lower arms, palms, and fingers.

7. Relax your chest, navel, lower abdomen, pelvis, and hips.

8. Relax your thighs, knees, calves, feet, ankles, and toes.

* This phase of the journey is a yoga nidra practice; you can do it on your own, as we've outlined here, or you can use an audio meditation, such as the one you'll find at www.awakenedsleep.net.

Phase 3: Invite Sattvic Awareness

1. With a feeling of restful awareness, gently think of your mantra that you use for your meditation practice. You can also use *Om Agasthi Shahina*—a mantra that embodies the essence of sattvic, awakened sleep.

2. Alternatively, you can use a mantra that corresponds to your dosha:
   a. Vata: *HREEM*, which is the seed mantra of prana, the heart, and movement
   b. Pitta: *SHREEM*, which is the seed mantra for cooling and soothing relaxation, as well as bringing calmness and tranquility

   c. Kapha: *KLEEM*, which is the seed mantra of the spiritual heart and of cultivating unconditional love and compassion

3. Keep repeating the mantra with deep, rhythmic breathing. You'll feel your body becoming heavy and relaxed, readying you for deep slumber and awakened sleep.

4. If you wake up in the middle of the night for any reason, return to your back, place awareness on the heart and the breath, and know that you'll be able to easily drift back to sleep.

Phase 4: Emerge into the Light

1. When you awaken in the morning, rub your palms and cover your eyes while taking deep breaths, expressing gratitude and joy. Repeat your mantra three times.

2. Get up and sit at the edge of your bed. Do a few neck and shoulder rolls/stretches.

3. Ask yourself three questions: *How good was my sleep? Do I feel rested, relaxed, and energized? Do I remember my dreams?*

4. Set an intention for your day.

5. Ready yourself for an awakened day.

SATTVIC RECIPES FOR AWAKENED SLEEP

On the following pages, we offer four specially chosen sattvic recipes crafted to support a calm state conducive to awakened sleep. While the world of sattvic foods is extensive—after all, Ayurveda offers highly specialized routines for the doshas, the seasons, and the specific imbalances we might be experiencing—we've selected these recipes specifically for their ability to promote a balanced, grounded quality—neither too heavy nor too light—that aligns with the Awakened Sleep Technique. Unlike foods that lead to a tamasic influence, which can dull awareness, these recipes foster a still, clear state of lucidity, setting the stage for a deeply restful and mind-expanding sleep experience. May they bring you closer to a night of nourishing, transformative rest.

CATCH THOSE Z'S: AN
HERBAL TRANQUILI-TEA

Davidson Organics offers a special line of Ayurvedic herbal teas, formulated by Dr. Suhas. This line includes a delightful sleep tea, crafted with a blend of powerful, organic ingredients to support deep, restorative sleep. This soothing tea combines chamomile flower and lavender flower, both known for their calming effects, with gotu kola leaf to promote relaxation. Orange peel, cinnamon bark, and cardamom seed add a warm, comforting flavor, while licorice root enhances the blend's natural sweetness. Together, these ingredients create a tea that aligns beautifully with Ayurvedic principles, balances all the doshas, and invites a restful night's sleep through the gentle power of nature.

If you're interested in making your own blend, we created the following soothing tea recipe to promote a restful sleep by balancing calming herbs with warming spices. It can be modified to balance your dosha imbalance, or according to the season.

Ingredients

1 part organic passionflower
1 part organic chamomile flower
1 part organic lavender flower
1 part organic lemon balm
½ part organic licorice root
½ part spice blend of organic cardamom, saffron, and cinnamon

Instructions

Prepare the ingredients: Combine each of the herbs and spices as listed, measuring them according to the proportions above. For ease, if using 1 tablespoon as "1 part," add 1 tablespoon each of passionflower, chamomile, lavender, and lemon balm; ½ tablespoon of licorice root; and ½ tablespoon of the spice blend.

Mix the herbs and spices: Place all ingredients in a bowl and gently mix to evenly distribute the herbs and spices.

Boil the water: Bring 2 cups of water to a gentle boil.

Steep the tea: Add 1–2 teaspoons of the tea blend to an infuser or directly into a teapot. Pour the hot water over the tea blend and let it steep for 5–7 minutes to fully release the flavors and beneficial properties.

Strain and serve: Strain the tea into a cup. Optionally, add a touch of honey if desired.

Enjoy: Sip slowly, about thirty minutes before bedtime, to promote relaxation and prepare for a peaceful, restorative sleep.

Storage

Store any remaining tea blend in an airtight container in a cool, dark place to preserve freshness.

SWEET DREAMS: GOLDEN MILK TO PACIFY YOUR SLEEP

Golden milk, known as *haldi doodh*, is a deeply soothing and nourishing Ayurvedic drink that helps calm the mind and body. It's a holistic remedy designed to promote digestion and ease the mind into a peaceful, restful sleep. Turmeric's anti-inflammatory properties support the body while synergizing with spices like cardamom, ginger, and black pepper to warm the system and soothe the digestive tract. Ashwagandha adds an adaptogenic quality, helping the body cope with stress and balance the nervous system, while saffron and nutmeg contribute to an overall sense of comfort and relaxation. The blend creates a warming, comforting quality that not only supports the body's natural ability to rest but also helps balance the doshas, especially Vata.

In the bustling, vibrant streets of India, where chaos and energy seem to buzz at every corner, there's a beautiful paradox that visitors often notice: Despite the hectic pace, there's a deep spiritual temperament of centering and balance. Golden milk has been a comforting tradition for generations, bringing a sense of peace amid the swirl of daily life. It's a reminder that even in the busiest moments, it's possible to find calm and return to a place of balance, inviting restful sleep and a peaceful state of mind—just like it has for countless people in India for centuries.

Ingredients

2–3 saffron threads (soaked in a little warm water)
½ teaspoon organic turmeric
¼ teaspoon organic ginger (ground)
½ teaspoon organic ashwagandha powder
Pinch of black pepper (to activate turmeric's benefits)
¼ teaspoon organic cardamom

Pinch of organic nutmeg

1 cup full-fat milk (dairy or plant-based like coconut or almond milk)

1–2 pitted dates (or to taste, for sweetness)

1 teaspoon coconut sugar (optional, for added sweetness)

Instructions

Prepare the saffron: Begin by soaking the saffron threads in a small bowl of warm water for five minutes. This helps release the full flavor and healing properties of the saffron.

Combine the dry ingredients: In a small saucepan, place the turmeric, ginger, ashwagandha, black pepper, cardamom, and nutmeg. Stir gently to combine the spices.

Add milk: Pour the milk of your choice into the saucepan with the dry ingredients. Use medium heat, and gently stir the milk as it warms, allowing the spices to blend.

Sweeten the milk: Add the soaked saffron (with its water), pitted dates, and coconut sugar (if using). Continue to stir until the dates dissolve completely, the milk becomes golden in color, and the mixture reaches a gentle simmer.

Simmer: Let the milk simmer for five to seven minutes, allowing the flavors to fully infuse the milk. Be careful not to let it boil over.

Strain and serve: Once the golden milk has reached a smooth, creamy consistency, strain it into your favorite mug to remove any remaining spice particles.

Enjoy: Sip slowly, about thirty minutes before bed. As you drink, focus on letting go of the day's stimuli, feeling the warmth of the milk nurturing you back to the peaceful, restful state of sleep.

SUPERFOOD FOR SLUMBER: KHICHADI

Khichadi is a deeply nourishing, easy-to-digest dish that has been a cornerstone of Ayurvedic cooking for centuries. The simple combination of rice, split mung beans, and warming spices provides a perfect balance of proteins, carbohydrates, and fats. Known for its detoxifying and grounding properties, khichadi is especially beneficial as a light evening meal. The combination of slowly released carbs and gentle spices helps to stabilize blood sugar, promote relaxation, and prepare the body for sleep. Soothing spices, including turmeric and coriander, promote digestion and reduce inflammation. The natural amino acids in mung beans also encourage the production of serotonin—a key precursor to melatonin, the sleep hormone. The addition of coconut milk and ghee gives you healthy fats that stabilize energy levels, making it easier to unwind and drift into restorative sleep. Its ease of preparation and versatility make khichadi an ideal healthy dinner option for busy evenings or times when you need something light yet satisfying.

Ingredients

1 cup white basmati rice, rinsed thoroughly
½ cup split mung dahl (split hulled mung beans), rinsed
3 cups filtered water
1 zucchini, chopped / leafy greens, chopped / peas (vegetables of choice)
1 small sweet potato, peeled and chopped (optional)
2 teaspoons curry powder or garam masala (an Indian all-spice blend)
2 tablespoons lemon juice
Salt, to taste
Freshly ground black pepper
Fresh cilantro, for garnish
Ghee, for garnish

Instructions

In a medium saucepan, combine the rinsed rice, mung dahl, and water. Bring to a boil over high heat.

Reduce the heat to low, cover, and simmer for ten minutes.

Add an even layer of vegetables on top of the rice mixture without stirring. Cover again and continue to cook for about twenty minutes, or until the rice mixture has absorbed all the water.

Once the rice mixture is cooked, stir in the curry powder and lemon juice. Simmer briefly until all the liquid is absorbed and the dish is creamy.

Season with salt and freshly ground black pepper to taste.

Garnish with fresh cilantro and a drizzle of ghee. Serve immediately.

MODIFY YOUR ROUTINE FOR THE DOSHAS

Refer to the assessment from Chapter 1 (What Kind of Sleeper Are You?, page 40) to find your prakruti (the dosha or natural constitution with which you were born) and the assessment from Chapter 2 (Which Dosha Is Keeping You Up at Night?, page 70) to find your vikruti (an imbalance in your natural constitution based on your lifestyle and other circumstances). Then, based on both of these, check out the dosha-balancing tips that follow, which can be used to round out your daily routine.

Vata

- In your bath, shower, or an aromatherapy diffuser, use essential oils such as basil, lavender, orange, geranium, clove, and rose, which calm and settle down restlessness and quiet the mind.
- Consider alternate-nostril breathing for additional grounding and balancing of the nervous system.
- For self-massage, use a grounding oil, such as sesame or almond.

Pitta

- In your bath, shower, or an aromatherapy diffuser, use essential oils such as sandalwood, mint, lavender, jasmine, and vetiver, which are cooling and sweet and can help to release hostile emotions and regulate heat.
- Consider ujjayi breathing to tone the vagus nerve and reduce inflammation in the body and mind.
- For self-massage, use a cooling oil, such as coconut, with a few drops of sandalwood essential oil.

Kapha

- In your bath, shower, or an aromatherapy diffuser, use essential oils such as ginger, eucalyptus, menthol, camphor, clove, and juniper, which have a decongesting effect and help to combat water retention and other blockages in the body.
- Consider ujjayi breathing to calm yourself before bed.

- For self-massage, use a warming oil, such as sunflower, safflower, or mustard oil. For extra invigoration, you can also try dry brushing—use a brush with soft bristles on dry skin.

REFLECTIONS

1. How do you currently go to sleep each night, and what thoughts or habits typically fill your mind right before bed?
2. How do you usually wake up in the morning, and how does this affect the rest of your day?
3. How would you like to go to sleep, and what changes could you make to create a calmer, more peaceful transition into rest?
4. How would you like to wake up, and what morning rituals can you incorporate to set a positive tone for your day?
5. How can you ritualize sleep for your partner or family to create a shared sense of calm and connection in the evenings?
6. Reflecting on the five-senses therapy we explored in Chapter 5, craft a nightly routine that engages each of your senses to promote relaxation and restfulness. Personalize your nighttime routine based on Ayurvedic principles, considering your unique dosha and lifestyle needs.

CRAFT YOUR OWN EVENING ROUTINE

Just as you did in Chapter 9, revisit the assessment in Chapter 3 (Your Dosha Clock—Time Your Perfect Day, page 102), which you can use as a reference to create a more comprehensive evening/nighttime routine for your dosha.

On the following pages, we include Moira's nighttime routine.

Time of Day	Dominant Dosha	Activities
6–7 p.m.	Kapha	Finish with dinner and dishes; ask kids to help. Do some light journaling if I didn't before dinner.
7–8 p.m.	Kapha	Help kids with homework. Eliminate TV and background noise. Leave our gadgets on the dining room table.
8–9 p.m.	Kapha	Get kids to bed. Perform bathroom routine: shower with some aromatherapy (currently a combination of lavender and rose to balance both Vata and Pitta). Brush teeth.
9–10 p.m.	Kapha	Massage scalp, ears, and feet with my favorite coconut oil–based body oil to balance excess Pitta during this transitional time of life. Do a five-minute breathwork practice.
10–11 p.m.	Pitta	Get comfortable under my weighted blanket. Alternate between yoga nidra practice and Awakened Sleep Technique at 10 p.m. before drifting into sleep.
11 p.m.–12 a.m.	Pitta	Sleep.
12–1 a.m.	Pitta	Sleep.
1–2 a.m.	Pitta	Sleep.
2–3 a.m.	Vata	If I wake up to go to the bathroom or with thoughts or dreams, do a brief yoga nidra / progressive relaxation technique.
3–4 a.m.	Vata	Sleep.
4–5 a.m.	Vata	Sleep.
5–6 a.m.	Vata	Wake up around 6 and move into morning routine with ease.

Now, it's time to create your own personalized routine from the suggestions in this chapter:

Time of Day	Dominant Dosha	Activities
6–7 p.m.	Kapha	
7–8 p.m.	Kapha	
8–9 p.m.	Kapha	
9–10 p.m.	Kapha	
10–11 p.m.	Pitta	
11 p.m.–12 a.m.	Pitta	
12–1 a.m.	Pitta	

Time of Day	Dominant Dosha	Activities
1–2 a.m.	Pitta	
2–3 a.m.	Vata	
3–4 a.m.	Vata	
4–5 a.m.	Vata	
5–6 a.m.	Vata	

CONCLUSION

) ▶ ● ◀ (

Sleep is the best meditation.

—His Holiness the Dalai Lama

A S WE REACH THE END OF OUR JOURNEY TOGETHER, IT'S IMPORTANT
to remember that sleep is not just a break from the demands of the
day—it is a sacred, spiritual opportunity that can deeply enrich your life,
even in the midst of the stressors and complexities of modern life. We
know that the pace of life today can feel overwhelming, and the challenges we face in balancing work, family, and spiritual pursuits are very
real. Yet, even amidst all the distractions and demands of contemporary
living, you have the power to make small changes that can transform
your sleep—and, ultimately, your life.

The wisdom of the ancients, particularly through the lens of Ayurveda,
offers timeless insights into how sleep can become more than a physical
necessity. It can be a gateway to a deeper connection with your true self,
your desires, and the universe. By understanding sleep as a mystical experience, you can begin to shift your perception, not as an escape from the
stress of the day but as a doorway to your highest potential. The physical
laws of the world may dominate your waking hours, but in sleep, the
boundaries dissolve, and you are free to explore new dimensions of your
being, which can enhance your experience of the waking world.

You may feel that sleep, at times, is elusive, or perhaps it's been clouded by stress, anxiety, or the weight of daily responsibilities. But know this: Even small adjustments in how you approach sleep can yield profound changes. Begin with the basics: Create a rhythmic, calming routine around your sleep. Allow yourself to gradually disconnect from screens, work, and any distractions that rob you of rest. Let sleep be a sacred time during which you slow down the rhythm of your being in a way that nurtures your soul and prepares you for the challenges of the day ahead.

In this space of rest, you can connect with the silence, the gap between thoughts, and the timelessness that is so rare in our busy lives. You don't need to be perfect or have all the answers. Just like the patients whose stories we've shared, you can simply take steps to honor this time; seeking out the quiet moments of peace will help you begin to plant seeds of transformation. Through these practices, you will begin to tap into the field of pure potentiality, where your dreams, desires, and intentions can take root. Even if it's just a few minutes of conscious relaxation or a slight shift in your evening habits, know that you are making a difference.

Deep, awakened sleep is within your reach. It doesn't require perfection, just presence. With the nurturing guidance of Nidra Devi, the goddess of sleep, you can start to experience a sleep that is not just restful but deeply restorative. This isn't about escaping the challenges of life, but rather transforming them through your connection to the wisdom of the ages and the potential within you.

As you close this book, know that the tools and practices shared here are not beyond your reach. You don't need to make huge changes overnight. The ancient teachings of Ayurveda and the sacred rituals of sleep can be adapted to fit your life, no matter how busy or complicated it may feel. Take it one step at a time. With patience, compassion, and a little consistency, you can begin to tap into the profound power of sleep—and awaken to the deepest parts of yourself, one peaceful night at a time.

Sleep is like a lamp at the door, giving you a glimpse into your consciousness, illuminating both your inner world and the world around
you. It's a chance to heal and awaken to the deeper truths of your existence. While sleep is often associated with darkness and fear, it doesn't
have to be. These feelings can be dispelled with practice. The techniques
shared in this book are designed to help you convert sleep into something
better—something to look forward to. When you approach sleep with a
peaceful, sattvic quality, it becomes a tool for self-discovery.

Throughout the day, sensory stimulation and emotional stress churn
the waters of your mind. But in the stillness of sleep, these disturbances
slow down, allowing you to see what's coming to the surface. In this
way, sleep becomes a powerful catalyst for changing your life. For sleep
is where you move beyond the physical laws that govern our waking lives
and become part of the ever-expanding consciousness that pervades the
universe. Sleep becomes an opportunity to witness your place within that
vast, universal flow, accessing knowledge beyond your habitual thoughts.

In sleep, you connect with Shakti, the creative energy behind all of
creation. Mother Nature, in her infinite wisdom, guides you to a know-
ingness that is ingrained in nature itself. Sleep is not simply a biological
necessity—it's a key to a healthier, more peaceful, and more awakened
life. It's a gift you give to yourself every night, one that can transform
your world when you choose to approach it with reverence, mindfulness,
and gratitude.

We leave you with the translation of a beautiful prayer from the *Devi
Mahatmya*, a text that celebrates the love and power of the divine femi-
nine in all her forms. This prayer is known as the *Ratri Suktam*, or the
Hymn to the Goddess of Night. The hymn is a testament to the ways
in which we can dispel the darkness of ignorance even as we enter the
depths of sleep and make contact with another glorious goddess, Yoga
Nidra. Here, we enter into a different kind of darkness: the womb of
sleep, in which all things are possible and we can dive into the ocean of

consciousness. Feel free to use this hymn, which we have reimagined to evoke the essence of its powerful message, as a contemplation to guide you in the transition between wakefulness and sleep. Rather than being a literal translation, our version captures the spirit of the original, reflecting the dance of consciousness and the journey into awakened sleep. Let it inspire you as you cross the threshold into expanded awareness—the gateway to self-realization.

> *O Ratri, goddess of the night,*
> *You spread your veil over the world,*
> *A blanket of peace,*
> *Where all is held in your loving care.*
> *You nurture the universe with your gentle presence,*
> *Every living being finds refuge in your embrace,*
> *And in the stillness of the night,*
> *The seeds of creation are nourished.*
> *You are the keeper of the balance,*
> *Between the light and the dark,*
> *Between ignorance and knowledge,*
> *Guiding the soul through the depths of sleep,*
> *And awakening it with the dawn of wisdom.*
> *In the quiet of dusk,*
> *In the clarity of dawn,*
> *We feel the pulse of your wisdom,*
> *The rhythm of the cosmos,*
> *The underlying intelligence of creation.*
> *O Nisha, you are the darkness that holds us,*
> *O Usha, you are the light that illuminates our path.*
> *Together, you are the eternal dance,*
> *The play of the gunas,*
> *Sattva, Rajas, and Tamas,*

The forces that shape the world
And move through every moment.
In your embrace, we remember,
The truth of our being,
The truth of the universe,
That we are not bound by time or form,
But are eternal,
Part of the great cycle of creation,
Preserved and nurtured by your grace.
O Ratri, goddess of the night,
You are the mother of all,
The source of all wisdom,
The intelligence that flows through every thought,
Every sound, every movement.
In your silence, we find our voice,
In your stillness, we find our truth.

ACKNOWLEDGMENTS

Dr. Suhas Kshirsagar

As I reflect upon my life so far, I can express my sincere thanks and heartfelt gratitude to so many people who have inspired and illuminated my path. A big thank-you to all my patients and students who bestowed their trust in me for their own wellness journey. Today, I greatly miss my parents, Govind and Shalini, who instilled the core values of hard work, discipline, and courage in me. They always encouraged me to explore new frontiers. To my lovely wife, Dr. Manisha, who made our turbulent life look so easy and effortless. She is a true gift who has made all our lives truly abundant. As we traveled around the globe, she quietly raised our beautiful children, Manas and Sanika, who have blossomed as smart health care professionals and have found perfect partners in Vallari and Srikar. Our extended family has brought so much love and happiness into our lives. As we expect our first grandchild this year, we feel truly blessed for this wonderful life.

I would like to express deepest gratitude to my guide, mentor, and dear friend Dr. Deepak Chopra, who has been an inspiration behind all my books. His unwavering support and guidance are greatly appreciated. He is a master at what he does, and I feel blessed to have learned from the very best.

I am forever in debt to His Holiness Maharishi Mahesh Yogi, the founder of the Transcendental Meditation Movement, who gave me a glimpse of cosmic reality and taught me the modern-day application of Vedic sciences.

My coauthor, Dr. Sheila Patel, is a wonderful human being who has enriched this book with her insightful wisdom. It was so much fun and easy to work with her gracious smile and positive attitude.

A big thanks to our brilliant writer Nirmala Natraj, who effortlessly blended Ayurveda and modern science with her razor-sharp ability.

My book agent, Amanda Annis at Trident Media, is an anchor to many of my projects. I deeply value her guidance. A heartfelt thank-you to our publishing team at Grand Central Publishing, especially to our editor, Nana Twumasi. She believed in and supported this project from the very beginning. A big thanks to the Hachette team including Natalie Bautista; Cisca Schreefel; Terri Sirma, who created the beautiful book cover; and Amy Quinn, who made the layout so attractive.

My staff at Ayurvedic Healing has been a solid rock to anchor all my travels and changing schedules. A big thank-you to the entire Chopra family of teachers and educators. I am very fortunate to have received tremendous support from my Ayurveda fraternity, including Drs. Vasant Lad, David Frawley, and John Douillard.

All my books and travels have provided me a precious opportunity to look back and ponder my own journey from rural India, along many continents to a perfect landing in the US. Along my path, countless hands, guides, and mentors have shared their love and wisdom with me, and I express my sincere gratitude to each one of them.

Dr. Sheila Patel

My participation in writing this book would not have been possible without the support and encouragement of a large community of family, friends, colleagues, and teachers, and I am grateful to each and every one. And, of course, a special thank-you to Dr. Deepak Chopra for being the inspiration behind bringing this book to life.

I never imagined I would write a book. My work typically happened within the privacy of four walls. But so much of my own inspiration and learning came from books, and Ayurveda itself inspired me to share these life-changing teachings through speaking and writing. The principles made sense to me, and the practices healed so many issues that medicine couldn't. As I began to live an Ayurvedic lifestyle, I realized how important sleep was to my own health. I was told that I had a condition called "dry eyes" as a teen and that I was "just a headache person" as an adult, so it fascinated me that by following the principles of Ayurveda (going to bed at a regular time and using the practices that we share in this book), these "lifelong" conditions could disappear, and my body could heal. And although I went through stages in life where sleep wasn't possible (being on call, working all night, or staying up all night with kids), I now know that awakened, healing sleep can be ours when the situation allows. And so, this book.

With that in mind, I would like to first thank my parents, Ambalal and (late) Sumitraben Patel, who served as my earliest spiritual guides and taught me to think openly and with curiosity. They instilled in me a deep appreciation for service to others, a guiding principle that I carried with me into my medical training. Above all else, their unconditional love and acceptance have always given me the courage and confidence to stay true to myself.

I would not be where I am today without the constant love and encouragement of my sister, Bhavana; my brother, Nehal; and my tribe of amazing friends. You all uplift me and keep me going.

Thank you to my children, Isaac and Sonya Brieske—you are my guiding lights on my path forward. Any healing I am able to offer the world is, in the deepest sense, for you.

I am grateful to my many teachers and mentors in medical school and residency who taught me the principles and practice of Western medicine. Without them, I would not have had the immense honor of caring for people who were critically ill and witnessing firsthand the power of modern medicine as well as the resilience of the human body, mind, and spirit.

I am especially grateful to the mentors who illuminated my path to Ayurveda: to Dr. Deepak Chopra and the late Dr. David Simon, who were my first teachers of Ayurveda, meditation, and yoga as whole-systems medicine and who imparted the profound wisdom of integrating both mind and heart in the care of patients. To Dr. Suhas Kshirsagar, my mentor, friend, and coauthor, who continually inspires me through his knowledge, wisdom, and humor. They have taught me the power of our innate healing abilities.

I am indebted to all the teachers—past, present, and future—who carry and pass on the knowledge of Ayurveda so that everyone can heal.

I am immensely grateful to the entire Chopra community, including certified Chopra teachers and coaches, guests at Chopra programs, and my many colleagues over the years at the Chopra Center and at Chopra Global. These shining lights brought Ayurveda to life and made it all fun.

I also must thank my coworkers in medicine over the years who sacrificed many hours of sleep in the service of others. Their dedication to our patients kept me going on those long, sleepless nights.

This book would not have been possible without the brilliant writing skills of Nirmala Nataraj. She was able to seamlessly weave together our varied experiences while bringing the voices of science and spirituality together.

Thank you to Amanda Annis and the team at Trident Media for your encouragement and guidance and for immediately believing in, and seeing the potential in, this book.

Thank you to Nana Twumasi and the team at Hachette publishing for taking us to the finish line.

Most important, I offer heartfelt thanks to all the patients I have had the privilege to serve—their stories have been among my greatest teachers, and I am deeply honored to have been a part of their healing journeys.

RESOURCES

The journey to awakened sleep doesn't end here—it's a lifelong exploration of health, balance, and expanded awareness. To support you in deepening your practice, we've curated a list of trusted resources from experts in Ayurveda, sleep science, and holistic health. Whether you're seeking practical sleep tips, transformative therapies, or spiritual insights, these tools and guides complement everything you've learned in this book and empower you to create a restorative and awakened sleep experience.

Awakened Sleep (www.awakenedsleep.net)

Your guide to embracing sleep as a mystical and transformative experience, this site complements the insights from *Awakened Sleep* with additional tools, meditations, recipes, and other resources to deepen your practice.

Dr. Suhas Kshirsagar (www.ayurvedichealing.net)

Dr. Suhas's website is a resource for Ayurvedic consultations, treatments, products, and tools to balance the body and mind, with a focus on lifestyle and dietary practices for restorative sleep. Here, you can also purchase Dr. Suhas's bestselling books: *Change Your Schedule, Change Your Life*; *The Hot Belly Diet*; and *Panchakarma*.

Dr. Sheila Patel (www.drsheilapatel.com)

Dr. Sheila is renowned for her expertise in integrative medicine, blending the wisdom of Ayurveda, meditation, and yoga with modern medical practices. She shares her perspectives on an Ayurvedic approach to health through her blog articles and shares ways to stay connected with her.

The Gaja Collective (www.thegajacollective.com)

The Gaja Collective is the home for Chopra courses, certifications, community, and educator support. It is ancient wisdom made practical and explored together, in community, to create lives of peace, health, and purpose.

Chopra Foundation (www.choprafoundation.org)

The Chopra Foundation is a nonprofit organization dedicated to improving health and well-being, expanding consciousness, and promoting world peace. It focuses on mind–body spiritual healing, education, and research, supporting initiatives such as empowering at-risk children, providing prenatal support, teaching meditation to prisoners, and advancing scientific studies on mind–body practices—all for the purpose of promoting a more peaceful and conscious world.

Ziva Health (www.ziva.health)

Ziva Health is an integrated health program that strives to transform wellness and health care through AI insights, real-time data, and cutting-edge tools that enable personalized, proactive care, including personalized sleep guidance.

National Sleep Foundation (www.thensf.org)

A reliable source for basic sleep hygiene, medical sleep disorders, and practical tips for improving sleep. Includes advice on mattresses, pillows, and daily routines.

Sleep Education (www.sleepeducation.org)

Provided by the American Academy of Sleep Medicine (AASM), this site offers in-depth patient information on sleep health, disorders, and therapies.

CBT-I Directory (www.cbti.directory)

An international directory of certified cognitive behavioral therapy for insomnia (CBT-I) therapists, this is a useful resource for addressing chronic sleep issues through evidence-based strategies.

iRest Institute (https://shop.irest.org)

An evidence-based meditation practice based on the ancient tradition of yoga nidra and adapted to modern life.

Polyvagal Institute (www.polyvagalinstitute.org)

A nonprofit organization whose mission is to advance social communication and connectivity by offering education based on polyvagal theory, which is a new understanding of the mind–body system and offers new approaches to the treatment of trauma.

NOTES

Introduction

1. Jay Summer, "Gallup Poll Shows US Adults Are More Stressed and Sleep Deprived Than Ever Before," Sleep Foundation, May 14, 2024, www.sleepfoundation .org/sleep-news/gallup-sleep-stress-poll.

2. Jianghong Liu et al., "Childhood Sleep: Physical, Cognitive, and Behavioral Consequences and Implications," *World Journal of Pediatrics* 20, no. 2 (2024): 122–132, https://doi.org/10.1007/s12519-022-00647-w.

Chapter 1

1. "Noncommunicable Diseases," Fact Sheets, World Health Organization, accessed November 19, 2024, www.who.int/news-room/fact-sheets/detail /noncommunicable-diseases.

2. Cother Hajat and Emma Stein, "The Global Burden of Multiple Chronic Conditions: A Narrative Review," *Preventive Medicine Reports* 12 (December 2018): 284–293, https://doi.org/10.1016/j.pmedr.2018.10.008.

3. "'Depression: Let's Talk,' Says WHO, as Depression Tops List of Causes of Ill Health," News, World Health Organization, March 30, 2017, www.who.int/news /item/30-03-2017--depression-let-s-talk-says-who-as-depression-tops-list -of-causes-of-ill-health.

4. Erica Coe et al., "In Search of Self and Something Bigger: A Spiritual Health Exploration," McKinsey Institute, May 13, 2024, www.mckinsey.com /mhi/our-insights/in-search-of-self-and-something-bigger-a-spiritual-health -exploration.

5. Melissa M. Lane et al., "Ultra-Processed Food Exposure and Adverse Health Outcomes: Umbrella Review of Epidemiological Meta-Analyses," *BMJ* 384 (February 2024): e077310, https://doi.org/10.1136/bmj-2023-077310.

6. Donato F. Romagnolo and Ornella I. Selmin, "Mediterranean Diet and Prevention of Chronic Diseases," *Nutrition Today* 52, no. 5 (2017): 208–222, https:// doi.org/10.1097/NT.0000000000000228.

7. Hannah Binks et al., "Effects of Diet on Sleep: A Narrative Review," *Nutrients* 12, no. 4 (2020): 936, https://doi.org/10.3390/nu12040936.

8. Michael Gleeson et al., "The Anti-Inflammatory Effects of Exercise: Mechanisms and Implications for the Prevention and Treatment of Disease, *Nature Reviews Immunology* 11, no. 9 (2011): 607–615, https://doi.org/10.1038/nri3041.

9. University of California, "Putting Feelings into Words Produces Therapeutic Effects in the Brain," *ScienceDaily*, June 22, 2007, www.sciencedaily.com/releases/2007/06/070622090727.htm.

10. Andrea Zaccaro et al., "How Breath-Control Can Change Your Life: A Systematic Review on Psycho-Physiological Correlates of Slow Breathing," *Frontiers in Human Neuroscience* 12 (September 2018): 353, https://doi.org/10.3389/fnhum.2018.00353.

11. Xianlin Zou et al., "The Genetics of Human Sleep and Sleep Disorders," *Annual Review of Genomics and Human Genetics* 25, no. 1 (2024): 259–285, https://doi.org/10.1146/annurev-genom-121222-120306.

Chapter 2

1. Adam Wichniak et al., "Effects of Antidepressants on Sleep," *Current Psychiatry Reports* 19, no. 9 (2017): 63, https://doi.org/10.1007/s11920-017-0816-4.

2. Kelsie M. Full et al., "Associations of Late-Life Sleep Medication Use with Incident Dementia in the Atherosclerosis Risk in Communities Study," *Journals of Gerontology: Series A, Biological Sciences and Medical Sciences* 78, no. 3 (2023): 438–446, https://doi.org/10.1093/gerona/glac088.

3. Jun-Wei Zheng et al., "Association Between Alcohol Consumption and Sleep Traits: Observational and Mendelian Randomization Studies in the UK Biobank," *Molecular Psychiatry* 29, no. 3 (2024): 838–846, https://doi.org/10.1038/s41380-023-02375-7.

4. Caio Amaral et al., "Cannabis and Sleep Disorders: Not Ready for Prime Time? A Qualitative Review," *Journal of Clinical Sleep Medicine* 19, no. 5 (2023): 975–990, https://doi.org/10.5664/jcsm.10428.

5. Evan A. Winiger et al., "Cannabis Use and Sleep: Expectations, Outcomes, and the Role of Age," *Addictive Behaviors* 112 (January 2021): 106642, https://doi.org/10.1016/j.addbeh.2020.106642.

6. "Cognitive Behavioral Therapy," AASM Sleep Education, accessed December 3, 2024, https://sleepeducation.org/patients/cognitive-behavioral-therapy.

7. Rob Newsom and Alex Dimitriu, "Cognitive Behavioral Therapy for Insomnia (CBT-I): An Overview," Sleep Foundation, updated May 7, 2024, www.sleepfoundation.org/insomnia/treatment/cognitive-behavioral-therapy-insomnia.

8. Fiona C. Baker et al., "Sleep and Sleep Disorders in the Menopausal Transition," *Sleep Medicine Clinic* 13, no. 3 (2018): 443–456, https://doi.org/10.1016/j.jsmc.2018.04.011.

9. Vanessa Muñiz et al., "Clinical Hypnosis and Cognitive Behavioral Therapy for Hot Flashes: A Scoping Review," *Women's Health Reports* 6, no. 1 (2025): 1–20, https://doi.org/10.1089/whr.2024.0144.

10. Geoffrey Calvert, "Shift Work and Sleep," *NIOSH Science Blog*, October 5, 2016, Centers for Disease Control and Prevention, https://blogs.cdc.gov/niosh-science-blog/2016/10/05/shift-work-and-sleep.

11. Qi-Jun Wu et al., "Shift Work and Health Outcomes: An Umbrella Review of Systematic Reviews and Meta-Analyses of Epidemiological Studies," *Journal of Clinical Sleep Medicine* 18, no. 2 (2022): 653–662, https://doi.org/10.5664/jcsm.9642.

12. Danielle Pacheco and Carly Snyder, "Sleep Deprivation and Postpartum Depression," Sleep Foundation, updated March 7, 2024, www.sleepfoundation.org/pregnancy/sleep-deprivation-and-postpartum-depression.

13. Pablo Álvarez-García et al., "Postpartum Depression in Fathers: A Systematic Review," *Journal of Clinical Medicine* 13, no. 10 (2024): 2949, https://doi.org/10.3390/jcm13102949.

14. Sammy Dhaliwal et al., "Sleep When the Baby Sleeps? The Effect of Daytime Nap Behaviors on Postpartum Depression Severity: A Stress Buffering Hypothesis," *Sleep* 46, supp. 1 (May 2023): A274–A275, https://doi.org/10.1093/sleep/zsad077.0625.

15. Frances O'Callaghan et al., "Effects of Caffeine on Sleep Quality and Daytime Functioning," *Risk Management and Healthcare Policy*, no. 11 (December 2018): 263–271, https://doi.org/10.2147/RMHP.S156404.

16. Institute of Medicine, "Pharmacology of Caffeine," in *Caffeine for the Sustainment of Mental Task Performance: Formulations for Military Operations* (National Academy Press, 2001), 25–31, https://doi.org/10.17226/10219.

Chapter 3

1. Jaime K. Devine and Jutta M. Wolf, "Determinants of Cortisol Awakening Responses to Naps and Nighttime Sleep," *Psychoneuroendocrinology* 63 (January 2016): 128–134, https://doi.org/10.1016/j.psyneuen.2015.09.016.

2. Hassan S. Dashti et al., "Genetic Determinants of Daytime Napping and Effects on Cardiometabolic Health," *Nature Communications* 12, no. 1 (2021): 900, https://doi.org/10.1038/s41467-020-20585-3.

3. Oliver Cameron Reddy and Ysbrand D. van der Werf, "The Sleeping Brain: Harnessing the Power of the Glymphatic System Through Lifestyle Choices," *Brain Sciences* 10, no. 11 (2020): 868, https://doi.org/10.3390/brainsci10110868.

4. Jayandra J. Himali et al., "Association Between Slow-Wave Sleep Loss and Incident Dementia," *JAMA Neurology* 80, no. 12 (2023): 1326–1333, https://doi.org/10.1001/jamaneurol.2023.3889.

5. Aakash K. Patel et al., "Physiology, Sleep Stages," in *StatPearls* (StatPearls Publishing, last updated January 26, 2024), Bookshelf, National Library of Medicine, www.ncbi.nlm.nih.gov/books/NBK526132.

6. Marta Zaraska, "Unlocking the Riddle of REM Sleep," Medscape, June 5, 2023, www.medscape.com/viewarticle/992776#vp_3.

7. Yuri Panchin and Vladimir M. Kovalzon, "Total Wake: Natural, Pathological, and Experimental Limits to Sleep Reduction," *Frontiers in Neuroscience* 15 (April 2021): 643496, https://doi.org/10.3389/fnins.2021.643496.

8. Eileen B. Leary et al., "Association of Rapid Eye Movement Sleep with Mortality in Middle-Aged and Older Adults," *JAMA Neurology* 77, no. 10 (2020): 1241–1251, https://doi.org/10.1001/jamaneurol.2020.2108.

9. Daniel P. Windred et al., "Sleep Regularity Is a Stronger Predictor of Mortality Risk Than Sleep Duration: A Prospective Cohort Study," *Sleep* 47, no. 1 (2024): zsad253, https://doi.org/10.1093/sleep/zsad253.

10. Muhammad Adeel Rishi et al., "Daylight Saving Time: An American Academy of Sleep Medicine Position Statement," *Journal of Clinical Sleep Medicine* 16, no. 10 (2020): 1781–1784, https://doi.org/10.5664/jcsm.8780.

11. Darius J. Nazir et al., "Monthly Intra-Individual Variation in Lipids over a 1-Year Period in 22 Normal Subjects," *Clinical Biochemistry* 32, no. 5 (1999): 381–389, https://doi.org/10.1016/S0009-9120(99)00030-2.

12. Narimen Yousfi et al., "Investigating the Potential Link Between Lunar Cycle and Multiple Sclerosis Relapses: A Call for Further Studies," *Libyan Journal of Medicine* 18, no. 1 (2023): 2238354, https://doi.org/10.1080/19932820.2023.2238354.

13. Youri G. Bolsius et al., "The Role of Clock Genes in Sleep, Stress and Memory," *Biochemical Pharmacology* 191 (September 2021): 114493, https://doi.org/10.1016/j.bcp.2021.114493.

14. Mégane Erblang et al., "Genetics and Cognitive Vulnerability to Sleep Deprivation in Healthy Subjects: Interaction of ADORA2A, TNF-α and COMT Polymorphisms," *Life* (Basel) 11, no. 10 (2021): 1110, https://doi.org/10.3390/life11101110.

15. Christian Jarrett, "Early Risers and Night Owls: A Neuroscientist Explains Who Is Happiest," Science Focus, BBC, November 20, 2023, www.sciencefocus.com/news/early-risers-and-night-owls-a-neuroscientist-explains-who-is-happiest.

16. Michael Breus, "Biphasic Sleep," Sleep Doctor, updated January 23, 2024, https://sleepdoctor.com/how-sleep-works/biphasic-sleep.

17. Ellen R. Stothard et al., "Circadian Entrainment to the Natural Light-Dark Cycle Across Seasons and the Weekend," *Current Biology* 27, no. 4 (2017): 508–513, https://doi.org/10.1016/j.cub.2016.12.041.

18. Punyakishore Maibam, "Role of the Ayurvedic Clock in Boosting the Immune System," *Journal of Ayurvedic and Herbal Medicine* 9, no. 2 (2023): 98–100, https://doi.org/10.31254/jahm.2023.9208.

19. Xin Tong and Lei Yin, "Circadian Rhythms in Liver Physiology and Liver Diseases," *Comprehensive Physiology* 3, no. 2 (2013): 917–940, https://doi.org/10.1002/cphy.c120017.

20. Sivarama Prasad Vinjamury et al., "Ayurvedic Therapy (Shirodhara) for Insomnia: A Case Series," *Global Advances in Health and Medicine* 3, no. 1 (2014): 75–80, https://doi.org/10.7453/gahmj.2012.086.

Chapter 4

1. American College of Cardiology, "Getting Good Sleep Could Add Years to Your Life," American College of Cardiology, press release, February 23, 2023, www.acc.org/About-ACC/Press-Releases/2023/02/22/21/35/Getting-Good-Sleep-Could-Add-Years-to-Your-Life.

2. Goran Medic et al., "Short- and Long-Term Health Consequences of Sleep Disruption," *Nature and Science of Sleep* 9 (May 2017): 151–161, https://doi.org/10.2147/NSS.S134864.

3. Roma Pahwa et al., "Chronic Inflammation," in *StatPearls* (StatPearls Publishing, last updated January 26, 2024), Bookshelf, National Library of Medicine, www.ncbi.nlm.nih.gov/books/NBK493173.

4. Michael R. Irwin et al., "Sleep Disturbance, Sleep Duration, and Inflammation: A Systematic Review and Meta-Analysis of Cohort Studies and Experimental Sleep Deprivation," *Biological Psychiatry* 80, no. 1 (2016): 40–52, https://doi.org/10.1016/j.biopsych.2015.05.014.

5. Mohammad A. Khan and Hamdan Al-Jahdali, "The Consequences of Sleep Deprivation on Cognitive Performance," *Neurosciences* (Riyadh) 28, no. 2 (2023): 91–99, https://doi.org/10.17712/nsj.2023.2.20220108; Rebecca F. Gottesman et al., "Impact of Sleep Disorders and Disturbed Sleep on Brain Health: A Scientific Statement from the American Heart Association," *Stroke* 55, no. 3 (2024): e61–e76, https://doi.org/10.1161/str.0000000000000453.

6. Jayandra J. Himali et al., "Association Between Slow-Wave Sleep Loss and Incident Dementia," *JAMA Neurology* 80, no. 12 (2023): 1326–1333, https://doi.org/10.1001/jamaneurol.2023.3889.

7. Cara C. Tomaso et al., "The Effect of Sleep Deprivation and Restriction on Mood, Emotion, and Emotion Regulation: Three Meta-Analyses in One," *Sleep* 44, no. 6 (2021): zsaa289, https://doi.org/10.1093/sleep/zsaa289.

8. Adrienne LaFrance, "Trolls Are Winning the Internet, Technologists Say," *The Atlantic*, March 29, 2017, www.theatlantic.com/technology/archive/2017/03/guys-its-time-for-some-troll-theory/521046.

9. Yanjun Ma et al., "Association Between Sleep Duration and Cognitive Decline," *JAMA Network Open* 3, no. 9 (2020): e2013573, https://doi.org/10.1001/jamanetworkopen.2020.13573.

10. Spencer Nielson et al., "Rested and Connected: An Exploration of Sleep Health and Loneliness Across the Adult Lifespan," *Sleep* 47, supp. 1 (May 2024): A319–A320, https://doi.org/10.1093/sleep/zsae067.0746.

11. Stuti J. Jaiswal et al., "Using New Technologies and Wearables for Characterizing Sleep in Population-Based Studies," *Current Sleep Medicine Reports* 10 (January 2024): 82–92, https://doi.org/10.1007/s40675-023-00272-7.

Chapter 5

1. Joshua R. Ehrlich, "Untreated Vision Loss as a Modifiable Dementia Risk Factor," *JAMA Ophthalmology*, ahead of print, September 19, 2024, https://doi.org/10.1001/jamaophthalmol.2024.3991.

2. Amir Baniassadi et al., "Nighttime Ambient Temperature and Sleep in Community-Dwelling Older Adults," *Science of the Total Environment* 899 (November 2023): 165623, https://doi.org/10.1016/j.scitotenv.2023.165623.

3. Charlie Zhong et al., "Disparities in Greenspace Associated with Sleep Duration Among Adolescent Children in Southern California," *Environmental Epidemiology* 7, no. 4 (2023): e264, https://doi.org/10.1097/EE9.0000000000000264.

4. Jong Cheol Shin et al., "Greenspace Exposure and Sleep: A Systematic Review," *Environmental Research* 182 (March 2020): 109081, https://doi.org/10.1016/j.envres.2019.109081.

5. Bo Cui et al., "Effects of Chronic Noise on Glucose Metabolism and Gut Microbiota–Host Inflammatory Homeostasis in Rats," *Scientific Reports* 6 (November 2016): 36693, https://doi.org/10.1038/srep36693.

6. Susan Hurley et al., "Light at Night and Breast Cancer Risk Among California Teachers," *Epidemiology* 25, no. 5 (2014): 697–706, https://doi.org/10.1097/EDE.0000000000000137.

7. "68% of the World's Population Projected to Live in Urban Areas by 2050, Says UN," Department of Economic and Social Affairs, United Nations, May 18, 2020, www.un.org/uk/desa/68-world-population-projected-live-urban-areas-2050-says-un.

8. Andrea Zaccaro et al., "How Breath-Control Can Change Your Life: A Systematic Review on Psycho-Physiological Correlates of Slow Breathing," *Frontiers in Human Neuroscience* 12 (September 2018): 353, https://doi.org/10.3389/fnhum.2018.00353.

Chapter 6

1. Wei Bai et al., "Global Prevalence of Poor Sleep Quality in Military Personnel and Veterans: A Systematic Review and Meta-Analysis of Epidemiological

Studies," *Sleep Medicine Reviews* 71 (October 2023): 101840, https://doi.org/10.1016/j.smrv.2023.101840.

2. Monica Lewin et al., "Early Life Trauma Has Lifelong Consequences for Sleep and Behavior," *Scientific Reports* 9 (November 2019): 16701, https://doi.org/10.1038/s41598-019-53241-y.

3. Christa K. McIntyre, "Is There a Role for Vagus Nerve Stimulation in the Treatment of Posttraumatic Stress Disorder?," *Bioelectronics in Medicine* 1, no. 2 (2018): 95–99, https://doi.org/10.2217/bem-2018-0002.

4. Shuai Zhang et al., "Transcutaneous Auricular Vagus Nerve Stimulation for Chronic Insomnia Disorder: A Randomized Clinical Trial," *JAMA Network Open* 7, no. 12 (2024): e2451217, https://doi.org/10.1001/jamanetworkopen.2024.51217.

5. Adam Wichniak et al., "Effects of Antidepressants on Sleep," *Current Psychiatry Reports* 19, no. 9 (2017): 63, https://doi.org/10.1007/s11920-017-0816-4.

6. Julia Carbone and Susanne Diekelmann, "An Update on Recent Advances in Targeted Memory Reactivation During Sleep," *NPJ Science of Learning* 9 (2024), https://doi.org/10.1038/s41539-024-00244-8.

7. Autumn M. Gallegos et al., "Meditation and Yoga for Posttraumatic Stress Disorder: A Meta-Analytic Review of Randomized Controlled Trials," *Clinical Psychology Review* 58 (December 2017): 115–124, https://doi.org/10.1016/j.cpr.2017.10.004.

8. Joseph Walker III and Deborah Pacik, "Controlled Rhythmic Yogic Breathing as Complementary Treatment for Post-Traumatic Stress Disorder in Military Veterans: A Case Series," *Medical Acupuncture* 29, no. 4 (2017): 232–238, https://doi.org/10.1089/acu.2017.1215.

Chapter 7

1. Carl G. Jung, *Man and His Symbols* (Bantam Doubleday Dell, 1997).

2. Sophie Schwartz et al., "Enhancing Imagery Rehearsal Therapy for Nightmares with Targeted Memory Reactivation," *Current Biology* 32, no. 22 (2022): 4808–4816.e4, https://doi.org/10.1016/j.cub.2022.09.032.

3. Mrithunjay Rathore et al., "Functional Connectivity of Prefrontal Cortex in Various Meditation Techniques—a Mini-Review," *International Journal of Yoga* 15, no. 3 (2022): 187–194, https://doi.org/10.4103/ijoy.ijoy_88_22.

Chapter 8

1. Lisa Miller et al., "Neural Correlates of Personalized Spiritual Experiences," *Cerebral Cortex* 29, no. 6 (2019): 2331–2338, https://doi.org/10.1093/cercor/bhy102.

2. Michael J. Cooper and Maurice M. Aygen, "A Relaxation Technique in the Management of Hypercholesterolemia," *Journal of Human Stress* 5, no. 4 (1979): 24–27, https://doi.org/10.1080/0097840X.1979.10545991.

3. Seithikurippu R. Pandi-Perumal et al., "The Origin and Clinical Relevance of Yoga Nidra," *Sleep and Vigilance* 6, no. 1 (2022): 61–84, https://doi.org/10.1007/s41782-022-00202-7.

4. Bhalendu S. Vaishnav et al., "Effect of Yoga-Nidra on Adolescents Well-Being: A Mixed Method Study," *International Journal of Yoga* 11, no. 3 (2018): 245–248, https://doi.org/10.4103/ijoy.IJOY_39_17.

5. Romain Ghibellini and Beat Meier, "The Hypnagogic State: A Brief Update," *Journal of Sleep Research* 32, no. 1 (2023): e13719, https://doi.org/10.1111/jsr.13719.

6. Rollin McCraty and Maria A. Zayas, "Cardiac Coherence, Self-Regulation, Autonomic Stability, and Psychosocial Well-Being," *Frontiers in Psychology* 5 (September 2014): 1090, https://doi.org/10.3389/fpsyg.2014.01090.

Chapter 9

1. Girardin Jean-Louis et al., "Sleep Health and Longevity—Considerations for Personalizing Existing Recommendations," *JAMA Network Open* 4, no. 9 (2021): e2124387, https://doi.org/10.1001/jamanetworkopen.2021.24387.

INDEX

ABOUT THE AUTHORS

Together, Dr. Suhas Kshirsagar and Dr. Sheila Patel have taught and worked with more than one hundred thousand patients and clinicians for the purpose of bringing time-honored holistic healing practices to a Western audience. Through their unique and rigorous integrative approach, which combines Eastern and Western medicine and contemporary and ancient wisdom, Dr. Suhas and Dr. Sheila bring together empirical evidence, practical tools, and spiritual knowledge to empower people from diverse backgrounds to reap the benefits of taking their health into their own hands. As ancient wisdom practices continue to gain popularity, Dr. Suhas and Dr. Sheila are poised as experts who can offer readers accessible, actionable tools to change their lives from the inside out.

Dr. Suhas Kshirsagar (BAMS, MD, Ayurveda) is one of the most prominent and academically accomplished Ayurvedic physicians in the United States. He is the director of Ayurvedic Healing, an integrative wellness clinic in Santa Cruz, California, where he has successfully treated more than fifty thousand clients. He is also the author of *Change Your Schedule, Change Your Life* (Harper Wave, 2018), a book that has been translated into thirteen languages and sold more than forty thousand copies. As a leading voice in Ayurvedic medicine, Dr. Suhas is a sought-after speaker at Ayurvedic and wellness conferences, both nationally and internationally. He is an advisor and consultant at Chopra Global and Chopra Foundation, which allows him to share the stage with some of the leading global experts in the field of integrative medicine. These include Deepak Chopra, Andrew Weil, and Dean Ornish.

Dr. Suhas began his career in India, where he was classically trained in Ayurvedic medicine. He was a successful doctor in India when he received the call from His Holiness Maharishi Mahesh Yogi to join the transcendental meditation movement. Dr. Suhas and his wife, Manisha, spent more than twenty years traveling the world to teach wellness and meditation and to create Ayurvedic centers on every continent. During these years, Dr. Suhas saw the power of lifestyle changes with respect to optimizing personal health. He found that when people incorporated even a few dietary changes or tried meditation, yoga, and deep breathing, their lives transformed. This gave him the urge to teach. He eventually became the chairman of the Maharishi College of Vedic Medicine and a professor at the Maharishi International University. He served as the medical director of the Pancha-Karma Center in Fairfield, Iowa, before moving to Hawaii and later to California to begin his own wellness practice.

Currently, Dr. Suhas is a visiting faculty member at the Integrative Institute of Nutrition for their Health Coach training program. He serves as the Ayurvedic consultant and formulator for Vive Organic, Suja, Zrii, Davidson's Tea, Ayurvedic Infusions, Chopra products, Dr. Tung's, and other nutraceutical companies. He is on the board of directors of the National Ayurvedic Medical Association and the Association of Ayurvedic Professionals in North America and is a lead faculty member at Mount Madonna Institute, Sevanti Institute, and Kerala Ayurveda Academy in the United States.

Dr. Sheila Patel (MD) is a board-certified family physician who is passionate about bringing holistic healing practices into the Western medical system. After earning her MD at the University of Wisconsin School of

Medicine and Public Health, she completed her residency in family medicine at Ventura County Medical Center in California. For more than a
decade, she practiced full-spectrum family medicine (including prenatal care and deliveries, ER coverage, inpatient and outpatient care, and
end-of-life care). She practiced in small communities, first in Southeast
Alaska and then in rural Wisconsin, which allowed her to truly know
her patients. It was her patients who inspired her to continually learn,
look for answers, and find new tools for healing. This led her to pursue
education and training in other healing systems, including Ayurvedic
medicine. She currently maintains an outpatient primary care practice in
Southern California, where she combines the wisdom of ancient healing
traditions with the tools of modern medicine to help patients heal from
a variety of acute and chronic conditions. She is aware firsthand of the
challenges that patients face in the modern world and is passionate about
teaching patients practices to manage stress, get restful and rejuvenating
sleep, prevent chronic disease through healthy lifestyle, feel joyful and
purposeful, and truly thrive in their lives.

After completing her training in Ayurveda, Dr. Sheila served as the
medical director for Mind-Body Medical Group and the Chopra Center
for Wellbeing for ten years and then as chief medical officer for Chopra
Global. She is certified as an instructor of Ayurveda, yoga, and meditation and enjoys making these teachings accessible to all. She is currently
the chief medical officer for The Gaja Collective, where she is lead educator for the Chopra Ayurvedic health certification program. She is also
a faculty member at Yoga Veda Institute, where she teaches integrated
anatomy and physiology, bringing together concepts in Western medicine and Ayurveda. In addition, she has served as the clinical research
director for the Chopra Foundation, where she enjoyed shedding light on
the mechanisms of action of mind–body practices, giving them scientific
validation, and sharing this knowledge with others. She has coauthored
multiple published research papers on meditation and Ayurveda. Her

hope is that by confirming the benefits of the practices, more people will gain access to these life-enhancing techniques and shift the paradigm of healing to help people reach their full potential.

Dr. Sheila serves as a volunteer clinical faculty member at the University of California, San Diego, School of Family Medicine and Public Health, where she mentors medical students in primary care and integrative health to help train the next generation of physicians to bring true healing into medicine.

In addition to her work in health care, she is a sought-after keynote speaker, sharing her expertise in both conventional and traditional medicine with a variety of national and international audiences. Dr. Sheila is committed to supporting the expansion of knowledge of all healing practices and is dedicated to helping individuals achieve optimal health and well-being.

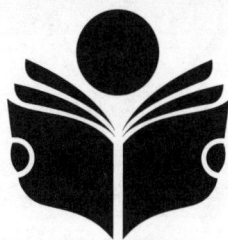

RAISING READERS
Books Build Bright Futures

Thank you for reading this book and for being a reader of books in general. As an author, I am so grateful to share being part of a community of readers with you, and I hope you will join me in passing our love of books on to the next generation of readers.

Did you know that reading for enjoyment is the single biggest predictor of a child's future happiness and success?

More than family circumstances, parents' educational background, or income, reading impacts a child's future academic performance, emotional well-being, communication skills, economic security, ambition, and happiness.

Studies show that kids reading for enjoyment in the US is in rapid decline:

- In 2012, 53% of 9-year-olds read almost every day. Just 10 years later, in 2022, the number had fallen to 39%.
- In 2012, 27% of 13-year-olds read for fun daily. By 2023, that number was just 14%.

Together, we can commit to **Raising Readers** and change this trend. How?

- Read to children in your life daily.
- Model reading as a fun activity.
- Reduce screen time.
- Start a family, school, or community book club.
- Visit bookstores and libraries regularly.
- Listen to audiobooks.
- Read the book before you see the movie.
- Encourage your child to read aloud to a pet or stuffed animal.
- Give books as gifts.
- Donate books to families and communities in need.

BOB1217

Books build bright futures, and **Raising Readers** is our shared responsibility.

For more information, visit **JoinRaisingReaders.com**

Sources: National Endowment for the Arts, National Assessment of Educational Progress, WorldBookDay.org, Nielsen BookData's 2023 "Understanding the Children's Book Consumer"